The Clinician's Guide to Common Psychiatric Disorders

Brooks Floyd • Timothy Kane

The Clinician's Guide to Common Psychiatric Disorders

A Pocketbook for Diagnosis and Treatment

Springer

Brooks Floyd
Comprehensive Behavioral Health
Staunton, VA, USA

Timothy Kane
Comprehensive Behavioral Health
Staunton, VA, USA

ISBN 978-3-031-67957-5 ISBN 978-3-031-67958-2 (eBook)
https://doi.org/10.1007/978-3-031-67958-2

This Springer imprint is published by the registered company Springer Nature Switzerland AG
The registered company address is: Gewerbestrasse 11, 6330 Cham, Switzerland

Preface

Being new at anything is very difficult. Being new to psychiatry sometimes seems insurmountable. That is how I felt when I started working in psychiatry 3 years ago. Even with nearly 15 years of healthcare experience, I was not ready for the complex field of psychiatry. Fortunately, for me, I was offered mentorship by Dr. Timothy Kane. Dr. Kane has over 30 years of experience in the field of psychiatry. He has worked in nearly every psychiatric setting including juvenile detention centers, prisons, hospitals, and private practice. He also published a psychopharmacology handbook used by the Federal Bureau of Investigation.

With a mentor like Dr. Kane, I listened intently and took notes to record all of the information I was exposed to on a daily basis. Eventually, these notes were converted into a resource I would provide my psychiatry students during their clinical rotations. The information packets received positive feedback, so I decided to publish the material to help others. That is how *The Clinician's Guide to Common Psychiatric Disorders* was born.

My hope is that this guidebook will assist providers new to the field of psychiatry to better understand how to treat common psychiatric disorders. I believe it can be used as a resource for primary care providers as well, as they are the first-line providers to those with mental health issues. What follows is the accumulation of 30 years of experience paired with an eagerness to help those overwhelmed by the field of psychiatry, just as I was 3 years ago.

Staunton, VA, USA — Brooks Floyd
Staunton, VA, USA — Timothy Kane

Acknowledgments

This book started as an idea to help new clinicians and Primary Care Providers ease into the often-puzzling world of psychiatry. I remember my first year as a Psychiatric Provider looking at the computer with a glazed look over my eyes wondering how I would ever be competent at prescribing medications. I want to thank Jaimie Smith for giving me the encouragement to pursue this endeavor, turn it into a book, and eventually attempt to get it published. Without her, this would still just be an idea.

I also want to thank my friend and supervising physician Dr. Timothy Kane who also co-authored this book. He was as about as supportive as an individual can be when I came to him with this project idea, and he gladly helped out whenever I asked. For that, I will be forever grateful.

I dedicate this book to my two daughters Olivia Grace Floyd and Ava Joelle Floyd. The two most important things to ever happen to me. Olivia was taken too soon and will be forever missed; I love you with all my heart. Ava has kept me going since Olivia's passing and is one of the reasons I am here to write this book. I love both of you unconditionally. I also want to thank my brother Mike Floyd for being there for me when times were and remain tough. Thanks brother.

Finally, I want to thank my favorite student that dealt with me trying to juggle writing a book, taking care of a full patient load, and still trying to squeeze in time to teach you in order to prepare you for your first year. Hopefully this book will be published in time to help you out.

Contents

Depressive Disorders

1

Contents

B. Floyd, T. Kane, *The Clinician's Guide to Common Psychiatric Disorders*, https://doi.org/10.1007/978-3-031-67958-2_1

Major Depressive Disorder (MDD)

Major depressive disorder is a mood disorder characterized by a persistent feeling of sadness, loss of interest, and/or anhedonia (lack of pleasure). Many people feel depressed throughout their lifetimes, but if symptoms are severe enough to interfere with daily life and last longer than 2 weeks, the person may be diagnosed with major depressive disorder.

Diagnosing and Monitoring

Mnemonic: Depressed Mood and Five or More Symptoms Lasting More Than 2 Weeks

SIGE-CAPS: **S**uicidal thoughts, **I**nterest decreased, **G**uilt, **E**nergy decreased, **C**oncentration decreased, **A**ppetite disturbance, **P**sychomotor agitation/retardation, **S**leep disturbances [1].

DSM-5-TR

The DSM-5-TR is used to diagnose major depressive disorder. In order to have an MDD diagnoses, you must have at least one of the first two symptoms listed and a total of five symptoms for more than a 2-week period. These symptoms are [2, p. 183] as follows:

- **Depressed mood**
- **Decreased interest/pleasure** in things you used to find interesting/pleasurable
- Decrease/increase in appetite nearly every day
- Insomnia/hypersomnia
- Psychomotor agitation/retardation
- Energy loss
- Decreased concentration
- Recurrent thoughts of death or suicide without a plan

Like all diagnoses in the DSM-5-TR, the illness should cause significant distress in the individual's life. Also, it cannot better be explained by a medical condition, substance, or other mental health disorder that would better explain the symptoms. There also must have never been a (hypo)manic episode. For a more comprehensive review, see the DSM-5-TR.

Differential Diagnoses: Adjustment disorder, persistent depressive disorder (dysthymia) bipolar disorder, cyclothymic disorder, schizophrenia, schizoaffective disorder, anxiety disorder, PTSD, delirium, substance use or withdrawal (alcohol, opiates, cocaine, cannabinoids, hypnotics), and personality disorders are associated with a higher risk of MDD but are likely aggravating factors rather than causative, medications (antihypertensives, steroids, chemotherapy), sleep-related disorders (OSA), endocrine disorders (hypothyroidism, Cushing disease, prolactinoma), infectious diseases (Lyme disease, mononucleosis, HIV, CNS syphilis), inflammatory conditions (SLE, multiple sclerosis), anemia, and Wilson disease.

Central nervous system diseases can produce a true depressive syndrome:
Parkinson disease
Dementia
Neoplasm
Huntington disease
Stroke
Epilepsy
B12 deficiency [3].

Risk Factors for Depression: Chronic medical illness, chronic daily stress, chronic pain, family history, female sex, job loss, low self-esteem, low social support, history of depression, single/divorced/widowed, TBI, younger age [4].

Labs to Consider: Complete blood count (CBC), complete metabolic panel (CMP) thyroid functioning tests, B12 levels, vitamin D, and folate levels. Urine drug screen if warranted. If the patient reports snoring, excessive daytime sleepiness, or apnea, consider sleep study.

Screening Scales

PHQ-9—It is a 9-question, self-administered diagnostic tool that rates the severity of depression based on the last 2 weeks. It takes less than 3 min to complete and is the most popular depression screener. Using a cut-off value of 10, it has a sensitivity and specificity of 85% and 85% [5].

HAM-D—It consists of 21 questions with only 17 being scored for severity of depression. It is clinician administered and more in depth while also being more time consuming than PHQ-9. It takes approximately 15 min to complete. Sensitivity and specificity values will vary based on the specific cutoff scores chosen for the HAM-D and the population being tested.

HAM-D6—It is an abbreviated 6-question, self-administered test. It can be completed in less than 3 min. The HAM-D6 has similar sensitivity to the HAM-D [6].

Quick Inventory of Depressive Symptoms (QIDS)—It is a 16-question, self-administered screener that is derived from the 9 DSM-V criteria for depression. Patient rates severity from 0 to 3. It has a sensitivity of 79% and specificity of 81% [7].

Beck Depression Inventory—It consists of 21 questions about how the patient has been feeling in the last week. It gauges depressive symptoms such as hopelessness and irritability and physical symptoms such as fatigue, weight loss, and lack of interest in sex.

Geriatric Depression Scale—It is a tool developed to help screen for depression in elderly patients. The traditional form consists of 30 questions while the short form consists of 15.

****The scale used is not as important as using the same scale consistently.****

Treatment

Psychotherapy response rate is approximately 40% and one third of depressed patients undergoing psychotherapy achieve remission [8]. Medication response rates vary depending on the source, but in the largest antidepressant trial to date, the Star-D trial showed remission rates ranging from 33% to 67%. Using a stepwise approach, the researchers developed an algorithm treatment approach that consisted of various antidepressants used in a stepwise manner. After one failure, they would proceed to step 2, then step 3, and so on. The Star-D trial showed that with persistent and vigorous medication management, those that were able to complete the study, remission was achieved as follows: about 33% after one step, 50% after two steps, 60% after three steps, and 67% after four steps. That still leaves approximately 30% of patients' depression unremitting and does not take into account those that stopped treatment due to unfavorable side effects [9].

The best approach for early sustained remission is a combination of psychotherapy and pharmacotherapy. For depression that is mild to moderate, psychotherapy has similar response rates to antidepressants. For severe depression, medication is first-line and combination therapy is warranted. MDD is a chronic, recurrent illness; the recurrence rate is about 50% after the first episode, 70% after the second episode, and 90% after the third episode which means some patients will require life-long medication therapy.

Non-pharmacologic Interventions

Cognitive Behavioral Therapy (CBT): It is a type of therapy that focuses on changing one's thoughts and behaviors to improve mood and functioning. It is a short-term, collaborative, goal-oriented therapy where the therapist helps the client identify negative thought patterns and behaviors and they develop ways to reconceptualize these thoughts and behaviors into something more positive. It is the most popular type of therapy for major depressive disorder.

Interpersonal Therapy (IPT): It is a type of therapy that focuses on interpersonal relationships and social interactions that can have an impact on your mental health. The therapist will help identify problem areas in the patient's relationships and outlines ways to address the difficulties which will in turn help alleviate depressive symptoms.

Acceptance and Commitment Therapy (ACT): It is a type of therapy where the patient accepts hardships and difficult emotions as they come and commit to making changes in their behavior that will positively impact their life regardless of the difficulties they have in their lives.

Relationships Matter

There is a growing body of evidence, that is, showing a patient's mental and physical health is greatly impacted by their social situation. Especially since COVID-19, many Americans are reporting increased levels of isolation and loneliness. Studies have shown that loneliness increases the risk of mortality similarly to those who smoke 15 cigarettes a day or someone who drinks 6 alcoholic beverages a day. Lack of social support and loneliness increases the risk of cardiovascular disease, type 2 diabetes, metabolic syndrome, and mild cognitive impairment/Alzheimer's disease and greatly raises relapse rates of depression once a patient has achieved remission.

It is imperative that we evaluate a patient's social support when we are evaluating their mental health. There is evidence that simple changes to lifestyle can have an effect size similar to antidepressant treatment. There are five changes a patient can make that will greatly increase their odds of achieving remission:

1. Exercise for 30 min a day, most days of the week. Any exercise that raises the heart rate is acceptable. Walking is a perfect low-cost activity to implement.
2. Practice mindfulness for 10 min a day, every day. There are free apps available to guide mindfulness meditation in most app stores.
3. Use 4 of the 6 sleep hygiene techniques to improve quality of sleep. These are as follows:
   (a) Turn off electronic devices 90 min before bed.
   (b) Avoid napping during the day.
   (c) Keep your bedroom as dark as possible.
   (d) Enjoy a warm, relaxing bath or shower before bed.

(e) Establish and stick to a regular bedtime each night.
(f) Avoid caffeinated drinks 10 h before bed.

4. Meet or call at least two family members or friends a day. Texting does not count.
5. Track daily meals, snacks, and drinks. Apps are available for this as well. The goal is to make small changes to improve your diet over time. Start by cutting out sugary beverages or snacks and replacing them with more nutritious food.

Studies show doing these five things consistently for 30 days will improve depressive symptoms similarly to taking an antidepressant alone. It is imperative that the patient not give up if they fail to do one of these things. Remind patients everyone makes mistakes, it is a process that over time will lead to significant changes in their lives. For more information you can visit: http://www.wild5wellness.com [10].

Treatment Recommendations for Major Depressive Disorder

First Line: Start Selective Serotonin Reuptake Inhibitor (SSRI): Escitalopram (Lexapro) and Sertraline (Zoloft) have best combination of efficacy and lowest side effect profile.

- If improvement is seen after 4–6 weeks, maximize dose.
- If there is no improvement after 4–6 weeks, change medication.
- If partial response and dose is maximized, add Bupropion (Wellbutrin).
- If side effects are intolerable, try another SSRI with comparable or better side effect profile.

Second Line: Try serotonin and norepinephrine reuptake inhibitor (SNRI)

- If modest improvement is seen after 4–6 weeks, maximize dose.
- If there is no improvement after 4–6 weeks, change medication and consider referral.
- If partial response and dose is maximized, add Bupropion (Wellbutrin) or consider atypical.
- If side effects are intolerable, try monotherapy Bupropion (Wellbutrin) or newer agents described below.

Third Line: Try newer agent such as Vilazodone (Viibryd), Vortioxetine (Trintellix), or (Dextromethorphan/Bupropion) Auvelity

- If improvement is seen after 4–6 weeks, maximize dose.
- If there is no improvement, augment with atypical antipsychotic and refer.
- If partial response and dose is maximized, add Wellbutrin or atypical plus referral.
- Refer to psychiatric specialist.

There are other available second- and third-line options such as lithium, but treatment-resistant patients should be managed by a seasoned psychiatric specialist.

First-Line Medications: SSRIs

Every SSRI and SNRI have the following black box warning: use may increase suicidal thoughts in children, adolescents, and young adults age 24 and younger. *Serious and life-threatening side effects underlined.*

Citalopram (Celexa)

Starting Dose: 20 mg PO daily. 10 mg PO daily can be used in elderly.

Titration: Increase to 40 mg PO daily—wait for 4–6 weeks for the response when initializing therapy.

Max Dose: 40 mg PO daily.

FDA Approval: Depression.

Common Side Effects: GI upset, sexual dysfunction, agitation, headache, bruising, and nausea, which should improve in 3–5 days.

Rare: *Seizures, hyponatremia, induction of mania, QTc prolongation, Serotonin Syndrome, bleeding, SIADH, and activation of suicidal ideation in those under 24.*

Monitoring: PHQ-9, ECG (if high risk or multiple QT prolonging medications), height and weight on children.

Contraindications: Taking MAO-I, pimozide, and known hypersensitivity to citalopram. Avoid in untreated angle-closure glaucoma.

Black Box Warning: Use may increase suicidal thoughts in children, adolescents, and young adults (24 and younger) [11].

Escitalopram (Lexapro)

Starting Dose: 10 mg PO daily. Can use 5 mg PO daily in Elderly.

Titration: Increase by 5–10 mg PO daily after 1 week. Wait for 4–6 weeks for the response when initializing therapy.

Max Dose: 20 mg PO daily.

FDA Approval: MDD (12 and up) and generalized anxiety disorder (GAD).

Common Side Effects: Fatigue, GI upset, sexual dysfunction, insomnia, bruising, agitation, headache, and nausea, which should improve in 3–5 days.

Rare: *Seizures, hyponatremia, induction of mania, Serotonin Syndrome, bleeding, SIADH, and activation of suicidal ideation in those under 24.*

Monitoring: PHQ-9, ECG if QT prolongation. Height and weight on children.

Pearl: Lexapro has the best side effect profile of all SSRIs.

Contraindications: Taking MAO-I, pimozide, and known hypersensitivity to escitalopram. Avoid in untreated angle-closure glaucoma.

Black Box Warning: Use may increase suicidal thoughts in children, adolescents, and young adults (24 and younger) [12].

Fluoxetine (Prozac)

Starting Dose: 20 mg PO daily. 10 mg PO daily can be used in elderly.

Titration: Increase by 20 mg PO daily after 1 week. Wait for 4–6 weeks for the response when initializing therapy.

Max Dose: 80 mg PO daily.

FDA Approval: MDD (8 and older), OCD (7 and older), PMDD, bulimia, panic disorder.

Common Side Effects: GI upset, sexual dysfunction, insomnia, anxiety, agitation, headache, dizziness, sweating, bruising, and nausea, which should improve in 3–5 days.

Rare: *Seizures, hyponatremia, induction of mania, Serotonin Syndrome, bleeding, SIADH, and activation of suicidal ideation in those under 24.*

Monitoring: PHQ-9, ECG if QT prolongation. Height and weight on children.

Pearl: No need to taper off medication when discontinuing due to long half-life.

Contraindications: Taking MAO-I, thioridazine, pimozide, and known hypersensitivity to Fluoxetine.

Black Box Warning: Use may increase suicidal thoughts in children, adolescents, and young adults (24 and younger) [13].

Paroxetine (Paxil)

Starting Dose:

Immediate Release: 20 mg PO daily. 10 mg PO daily can be used in elderly.

Controlled Release: 25 mg PO daily.

Titration:

Immediate Release: Increase by 10 mg PO daily, after 1 week. Wait for 4–6 weeks for the response when initializing therapy.

Controlled Release: 12.5 mg po daily, after 1 week. Wait for 4–6 weeks for the response when initializing therapy.

Max Dose:

Immediate Release: 50 mg PO daily.

Controlled Release: 62.5 mg po daily.

FDA Approval: MDD, OCD, Panic Disorder, SAD, PTSD, GAD, PMDD.

Common Side Effects: GI upset, sexual dysfunction, agitation, headache, sedation, dizziness, tremor, bruising, weight gain, and nausea, which should improve in 3–5 days.

Rare: *Seizures, hyponatremia, induction of mania, serotonin syndrome, bleeding, SIADH, and activation of suicidal ideation in those under 24.*

Monitoring: PHQ-9.

Pearl: There is a need to wean over several months for those who cannot tolerate withdrawal effects.

Contraindications: Taking MAO-I, pimozide, and known hypersensitivity to paroxetine.

Black Box Warning: Use may increase suicidal thoughts in children, adolescents, and young adults (24 and younger) ([14, 15].

*****Beers List for drugs to avoid in the elderly*****

Sertraline (Zoloft)

Starting Dose: 50 mg PO daily. 25 mg PO daily in elderly.

Titration: Increase by 25–50 mg PO daily every week. Wait for 4–6 weeks for the response when initializing therapy.

Max Dose: 200 mg PO daily.

FDA Approval: Major depressive disorder (MDD), obsessive compulsive disorder (OCD), panic disorder, posttraumatic stress disorder (PTSD), premenstrual dysphoric disorder (PMDD), social anxiety disorder.

Common Side Effects: GI upset, sexual dysfunction, agitation, headache, insomnia, sedation, sweating, bruising, and nausea, which should improve in 3–5 days.

Rare: *Seizures, hyponatremia, induction of mania, hypotension, Serotonin Syndrome, bleeding, SIADH, and activation of suicidal ideation in those under 24.*

Monitoring: PHQ-9.

Contraindications: Taking MAO-I, pimozide, and known hypersensitivity to Sertraline. Avoid in untreated angle-closure glaucoma.

Black Box Warning: Use may increase suicidal thoughts in children, adolescents, and young adults (24 and younger) [16].

SSRI-Like Medications

Vilazodone (Viibryd): SSRI Plus 5HT1A Partial Agonist

Starting Dose: 10 mg PO daily.

Titration: Increase by 10 mg PO daily every week. Wait for 4–6 weeks for the response when initializing therapy.

Max Dose: 40 mg PO daily.

FDA Approval: Major depressive disorder (MDD).

Common Side Effects: GI upset, sexual dysfunction, dry mouth, bruising, insomnia, dizziness, agitation, headache, and nausea, which should improve in 3–5 days.

Rare: *Seizures, hyponatremia, induction of mania, serotonin syndrome, bleeding, SIADH, and activation of suicidal ideation in those under 24.*

Monitoring: PHQ-9.

Pearl: It should be taken with food to aid in absorption.

Contraindications: Taking MAO-I. Avoid in untreated Angle-Closure Glaucoma.

Black Box Warning: Use may increase suicidal thoughts in children, adolescents, and young adults (24 and younger) [17]).

Vortioxetine (Trintellix): SSRI Plus 5H1 Receptor Modulator

Starting Dose: 10 mg PO daily. 5 mg PO daily in elderly.
Titration: Increase by 10 mg every week. Wait for 4–6 weeks for the response when initializing therapy.
Max Dose: 20 mg PO daily.
FDA Approval: Major depressive disorder (MDD).
Common Side Effects: GI upset, sexual dysfunction, and constipation.
Rare: *Seizures, hyponatremia, induction of mania, serotonin syndrome, and activation of suicidal ideation in those under 24.*
Monitoring: PHQ-9.
Contraindications: Taking MAO-I. Avoid in untreated angle-closure glaucoma.
Black Box Warning: Use may increase suicidal thoughts in children, adolescents, and young adults (24 and younger) [18].

SNRI Medications

Desvenlafaxine (Pristiq)

Starting Dose: 50 mg PO daily.
Titration: Increase by 50 mg PO daily. Wait for 4–6 weeks for the response when initializing therapy.
Max Dose: 400 mg PO daily.
FDA Approval: MDD.
Common Side Effects: INCREASED blood pressure, GI upset, sexual dysfunction, insomnia, dizziness, agitation, anxiety, sweating, headache, and nausea, which should improve in 3–5 days.

Rare: *Seizures, hyponatremia, induction of mania, serotonin syndrome, SIADH, and activation of suicidal ideation in those under 24.*

Monitoring: PHQ-9 and blood pressure at each visit.

Pearl: Higher doses are associated with more side effects.

Contraindications: Uncontrolled angle-closure glaucoma or taking a MAO-I.

Black Box Warning: Use may increase suicidal thoughts in children, adolescents, and young adults (24 and younger) [19].

Duloxetine (Cymbalta)

Starting Dose: 40 mg PO daily.

Titration: Increase by 20 mg PO daily first titration. Wait for 4–6 weeks for the response when initializing therapy. Then, it may be increased by 30 mg PO daily.

Max Dose: 120 mg PO daily.

FDA Approval: MDD, diabetic peripheral neuropathy, fibromyalgia, GAD, chronic musculoskeletal pain.

Common Side Effects: INCREASED blood pressure, GI upset, sexual dysfunction, insomnia, agitation, fatigue, dry mouth, sedation, sweating, dizziness, urinary retention, headache, blurred vision, and nausea, which should improve in 3–5 days.

Rare: *Seizures, hyponatremia, induction of mania, possible hepatotoxicity, orthostatic hypotension, Serotonin Syndrome, bleeding, SIADH, and activation of suicidal ideation in those under 24.*

Monitoring: PHQ-9 and blood pressure at each visit.

PEARL: Use may get benefit of pain reduction on 30 mg dose. It should be avoided with hepatic insufficiency.

Contraindications: Untreated angle-closure glaucoma, substantial alcohol use, taking a MAO-I, taking thioridazine.

Black Box Warning: Use may increase suicidal thoughts in children, adolescents, and young adults (24 and younger) [20].

Venlafaxine XR (Effexor XR)

Starting Dose: 37.5 mg PO daily.

Titration: Increase by 37.5 mg PO daily in 1 week. Then, titrate by 75 mg PO daily. Wait for 4–6 weeks (on 75 mg dose) for the response when initializing therapy.

Max Dose: 375 mg PO daily.

FDA Approval: Depression, GAD, SAD, panic disorder, separation anxiety disorder.

Common Side Effects: INCREASED blood pressure, GI upset, sexual dysfunction, insomnia, agitation, anxiety, sweating, abnormal vision, headache, and nausea, which should improve in 3–5 days.

Rare: *Seizures, hyponatremia, induction of mania, serotonin syndrome, SIADH, and activation of suicidal ideation in those under 24.*

Monitoring: PHQ-9 and blood pressure at each visit.

Pearls: Higher doses are associated with more side effects. Immediate release forms available but are more prone to discontinuation syndrome. Effexor can be difficult to wean; alternative strategies may need to be used and length of titration may take months. Patients commonly report "brain zaps" while discontinuing or even missing a dose. Medication is renally cleared and may need dose reduction of 25–50% in renal disease.

Contraindications: Uncontrolled angle-closure glaucoma or taking a MAO-I.

Black Box Warning: Use may increase suicidal thoughts in children, adolescents, and young adults (24 and younger) [21].

Adjunct Medications

Bupropion XL (Wellbutrin XL): Norepinephrine and Dopamine Reuptake Inhibitor (NDRI)

Starting Dose: 150 mg PO daily.

Titration: Increase by 150 mg PO daily. Wait for 4–6 weeks for the response when initializing therapy.

Max Dose: 450 mg PO daily.

FDA Approval: MDD, seasonal affective disorder, nicotine addiction (standard release).

Common Side Effects: Dry mouth, constipation, GI upset, insomnia, dizziness, headache, agitation, anxiety, tremor, sweating, weight loss, anorexia, myalgia, tinnitus, rash, and hypertension.

Rare: *Seizures, Stevens-Johnson syndrome has been reported, induction of mania, and activation of suicidal ideation in those under 24.*

Monitoring: PHQ-9 and blood pressure.

PEARL: XL only requires once a day dosing, making it the preferred preparation. It can be given with other antidepressants to help with sexual side effects.

Contraindicated: Patients with current or prior diagnosis of bulimia or anorexia nervosa. Patients with a history of seizures. If a patient is abruptly quitting alcohol, sedative use, or anticonvulsant medication. If a patient has had a recent head injury or has a nervous system tumor. If a patient is taking a MAO-I or Thioridazine.

Black Box Warning: Use may increase suicidal thoughts in children, adolescents, and young adults (24 and younger) [22].

Dextromethorphan/Bupropion (Auvelity): NDRI/NMDA Receptor Antagonist

Starting Dose: 45–105 mg PO daily.

Titration: Take 1 PO daily × 3 days and then take 1 PO twice daily. Take at least 8 h apart.

Max Dose: 90–210 mg PO daily.

FDA Approval: Major depressive disorder.

Common Side Effects: Dizziness, headache, somnolence, diarrhea, dry mouth, hyperhidrosis, and sexual dysfunction.

Rare: *Increased blood pressure, seizures, serotonin syndrome, psychosis, and induction of mania.*

Monitoring: PHQ-9 and blood pressure.

PEARL: It is the newest antidepressant on the market. It works as an NMDA receptors and can alleviate depression in 1 week compared to 4–6 weeks of traditional antidepressants.

Contraindicated: Patients with current or prior diagnosis of bulimia or anorexia nervosa. Patients with a history of seizures. If a patient is abruptly quitting alcohol, sedative use, or anticonvulsant medication. If a patient has had a recent head injury or has a nervous system tumor. Taking a MAO-I.

Black Box Warning: Use may increase suicidal thoughts in children, adolescents, and young adults (24 and younger) [23].

Mirtazapine (Remeron): Noradrenergic and Specific Serotonergic Antidepressant (NaSSA)

Starting Dose: 15 mg PO nightly.

Titration: Increase by 15 mg per titration.

Max Dose: Typically, 45 mg PO nightly.

FDA Approval: Major depressive disorder (MDD).

Common Side Effects: Dry mouth, constipation, weight gain, sedation, dizziness, confusion, urinary retention, abnormal dreams, hypotension, QTc prolongation, and flu-like symptoms.

Rare: *Agranulocytosis, serotonin syndrome, hyponatremia, seizures, induction of mania, and activation of suicidal ideation in those under 24.*

Monitoring: PHQ-9. EKG may be prudent if taking other QTc prolonging drugs, especially in the geriatric population.

PEARL: It is more sedating at lower doses with 7.5 mg being most sedating. It is often used for insomnia. Weight gain can be significant.

Contraindication: Patient taking a MAO-I.

Black Box Warning: Use may increase suicidal thoughts in children, adolescents, and young adults (24 and younger) [24].

Trazodone (Desyrel): Serotonin 2 Antagonist/ Reuptake Inhibitor (SARI)

Starting Dose: 150 mg in divided doses.

Titration: Increase by 50 mg PO nightly.

Max Dose: 400 mg PO daily.
FDA Approval: Major depressive disorder (MDD).
Common Side Effects: GI upset, sexual dysfunction, insomnia, agitation, sedation, dizziness, blurred vision, urinary retention, headache, nausea better in 3–5 days.
Rare: *Seizures, QTC prolongation, serotonin syndrome, hyponatremia, abnormal bleeding, orthostatic hypotension/syncope, hyponatremia, priapism, induction of mania, and activation of suicidal ideation in those under 24.*
Monitoring: PHQ-9. EKG may be prudent if taking other QTc prolonging drugs, especially in the geriatric population.
PEARL: It is often used for insomnia due to sedating properties at lower doses.
Contraindication: Patient taking a MAO-I.
Black Box Warning: Use may increase suicidal thoughts in children, adolescents, and youngadults (24 and younger) [25].

Atypical Antipsychotic Adjuncts

Aripiprazole (Abilify)

Starting Dose: 2–5 mg PO daily.
Titration: Increase by 2–5 mg PO daily every week.
Max Dose: 15 mg PO daily.
FDA Approval: Depression adjunct, schizophrenia, bipolar maintenance, autism-related irritability, Tourette's disorder in children ages 6–18, and agitation associated with schizophrenia or bipolar disorder (IM Abilify).
Common Side Effects: Dizziness, insomnia, akathisia, activation, nausea, vomiting, constipation, headache, orthostatic hypotension, tardive dyskinesia.
Rare: *Impulse control problems (gambling), hyperglycemia, neuroleptic malignant syndrome (NMS), seizures.*
Monitoring: PHQ-9, BMI every 3 months, lipid panel, and A1c annually. Waist circumference, blood pressure, fasting plasma glucose, and fasting lipid profile prior to start, within 3 months, and then annually. AIMS score every 3–6 months.

Pearl: Injectable form available.

Black Box Warning: Elderly dementia patients who take Abilify have a higher risk of death. Use may increase suicidal thoughts in children, adolescents, and young adults [26].

Brexpiprazole (Rexulti)

Starting Dose: 0.5–1 mg once daily.

Titration: May increase by 1 mg daily every week.

Max Dose: 3 mg PO daily.

FDA Approval: Treatment-resistant depression used as adjunct and schizophrenia.

Common Side Effects: Akathisia, weight gain, sedation, headache, and tardive dyskinesia.

Rare: *Impulse control problems (gambling), hyperglycemia, neuroleptic malignant syndrome, seizures.*

Monitoring: PHQ-9, BMI every 3 months, lipid panel, and A1c annually. Waist circumference, blood pressure, fasting plasma glucose, and fasting lipid profile prior to start, within 3 months, and then annually. AIMS score every 3–6 months.

Black Box Warning: Elderly dementia patients who take Rexulti have a higher risk of death. Use may increase suicidal thoughts in children, adolescents, and young adults (24 and younger) [27].

Cariprazine (Vraylar)

Starting Dose: 1.5 mg po daily.

Titration: Up to 3 mg after 14 days.

Max Dose: 3 mg.

FDA Approval: Schizophrenia acute and maintenance, acute mania/mixed mood, bipolar 1 (depression), MDD adjunct.

Common Side Effects: Akathisia, EPS, restlessness, GI distress, sedation, tardive dyskinesia.

Rare: *Hyperglycemia, neuroleptic malignant syndrome, and seizures.*

Monitoring: BMI monthly × 3 months then every 3 months. Blood pressure, fasting plasma glucose, fasting lipid panel within 3 months and then annually. More often if at risk for metabolic syndrome.

Pearl: Side effects may develop weeks later due to long half-life. 1.5 mg dose typically more effective for depressive symptoms.

Black Box Warning: Elderly dementia patients who take Vraylar have a higher risk of death. Use may increase suicidal thoughts in children, adolescents, and young adults [28].

Olanzapine-Fluoxetine (Symbyax)

Starting Dose: 6 mg/25 mg PO daily.

Titration: Increase by 3 mg of olanzapine or 25 mg of fluoxetine.

Max Dose: 18 mg/75 mg PO daily.

FDA Approval: Treatment-resistant depression, schizophrenia, bipolar maintenance, bipolar depression.

Common Side Effects: Increased risk of diabetes and dyslipidemia, dizziness, sedation, dry mouth, constipation, weight gain, edema, tachycardia, musculoskeletal pain, orthostatic hypotension, tardive dyskinesia.

Rare: *DRESS, hyperglycemia, neuroleptic malignant syndrome, and seizures.*

Monitoring: PHQ-9, BMI every 3 months, lipid panel, and A1c annually. Waist circumference, blood pressure, fasting plasma glucose, and fasting lipid profile prior to start, within 3 months, and then annually. AIMS score every 3–6 months.

Contraindications: Known risk of angle-closure glaucoma or unstable cardiac condition.

Black Box Warning: Elderly dementia patients who take Symbyax have a higher risk of death. Use may increase suicidal thoughts in children, adolescents, and young adults (24 and younger) [29]).

Quetiapine XR (Seroquel XR)

Starting Dose: 50 mg PO nightly.

Titration: Increase by 50 mg to 100 mg PO nightly every week.

Max Dose: Usually 300 mg PO daily for deression.

FDA Approval: MDD, bipolar depression, bipolar maintenance, schizophrenia.

Common Side Effects: GI upset, sexual dysfunction, insomnia, agitation, sedation, dizziness, urinary retention, headache, weight loss, myalgia, sweating, anorexia, hypertension, and nausea better in 3–5 days.

Rare: *Agranulocytosis, leukopenia, Neutropenia, Neuroleptic malignant syndrome, and seizures.*

Monitoring: PHQ-9, BMI every 3 months, lipid panel, and A1c annually. Waist circumference, blood pressure, fasting plasma glucose, and fasting lipid profile prior to start, within 3 months, and then annually. AIMS score every 3–6 months.

Pearl: It is known for its sedating properties and could be useful as an insomnia adjunct.

Black Box Warning: Elderly dementia patients who take Seroquel have a higher risk of death. Use may increase suicidal thoughts in children, adolescents, and young adults (24 and younger) [30].

Choosing Antidepressant Based on Comorbidities

Weight loss or loss of appetite	Remeron and Paxil
Weight gain	Wellbutrin
Insomnia	Remeron and trazodone
Hypersomnia	Wellbutrin, Cymbalta, Prozac, and Zoloft
Nerve pain/fibromyalgia	Cymbalta
Sexual dysfunction	Wellbutrin and mirtazapine [31]
Pregnancy	Zoloft (1st) and Lexapro. *Avoid Paxil*
Breastfeeding	Continue current antidepressant Zoloft and Paxil if medication naïve.

Traditional Medication Alternatives

The following therapies are not traditional antidepressants or augmentation strategies. They are typically reserved for treatment-resistant depression (TRD) and should be managed by a seasoned professional. Nevertheless, it is important that providers have a rudimentary understanding of alternative treatments in order to be a primer for their patient and briefly outline what these treatments entail. The following therapies are nontraditional, TRD alternatives: transcranial magnetic stimulation, Esketamine (Spravato), and electroconvulsive therapy (ECT).

Electroconvulsive Therapy (ECT)

Background: ECT has been in use since the 1920s but is being less frequently used due to the stigma surrounding it. ECT is the most efficacious treatment for depression that is available at this time. It also is the most invasive of all treatment options.

How it works: ECT involves a very complex mechanism of action that is not completely understood. Inducing a seizure seems to "reset" the brain and cause the release of chemicals related to mood regulation, quickly alleviating depressive symptoms.

Patient Experience: The patient will be placed on a stretcher in the procedure room. An IV will be inserted and the patient will have an oxygen mask placed. The patient will then be told to take deep breaths and an anesthetic will be given. The patient will fall asleep and the provider will use an electrode to deliver an electrical current to elicit a seizure. The patient will be unaware that anything has happened and will wake up in 5–10 min. They will be sleepy and possibly confused. They will be monitored in recovery for around 30 min and then released home. The patient is unable to drive for the day.

Side Effects: Nausea, muscle aches, jaw pain, headache, confusion, and retrograde amnesia. Increased risk of cardiac issues. Other side effects related to anesthesia risk are similar to minor surgeries.

Efficacy: Response rates are typically around 50% to 60% with some studies showing response rates as high as 75% [32].

Esketamine (Spravato)

Background: Spravato is an intranasal spray that was approved by the FDA in 2019 when used in conjunction with an antidepressant. It was the first NMDA receptor antagonist approved by the FDA. Spravato can only be delivered in Risk Evaluation and Mitigation Strategy (REMS) approved centers.

How It works: Esketamine, the S-enantiomer of racemic ketamine, works by blocking N-methyl-D-aspartate (NMDA) receptors which in turn increases levels of glutamate. Glutamate is a neurotransmitter that regulates learning and memory, but is also thought to play a role in mood regulation.

Patient Experience: The patient will be seated in a room by themselves in an REMS-approved center. Blood pressure will be taken at baseline. The patient will nasally inhale the medication in two sprays, one in each nostril. After 5 min, the patient will take the second dose totaling 58 mg. The patient may experience feelings of dissociation (being disconnected from one's thoughts), feelings of relaxation, and possible euphoria. There may be changes to visual perception as well. The patient will have their blood pressure taken a second time. The treatment lasts 2 h and the patient will not be allowed to drive after receiving treatment. Treatments are twice a week for 4 weeks and then once a week for 4 weeks, and maintenance is usually every other week with some people needing it weekly.

Side Effects: Temporary dizziness, confusion, lethargy, sedation, nausea, vomiting, difficulty urinating, and mild dissociation. Other possible side effects can include increased blood pressure and feelings of euphoria.

Efficacy: In a 2019 study, 69.3% of patients had a response to Spravato compared to 52% in the placebo group. 52.5% of patients achieved remission versus 31% in placebo [33].

Transcranial Magnetic Stimulation

Background: TMS is a noninvasive therapy that has been FDA approved for TRD since 2008. There is no medication involved although those on an antidepressant should continue their current medication regimen under the guidance of their prescriber.

How it works: TMS uses an electromagnetic coil that sends magnetic pulses to the left dorsolateral prefrontal cortex (LPFC), an area of the brain that is hypofunctional in depressed patients. The LPFC is thought to be the mood center of the brain and the magnetic waveforms used during TMS stimulate nerve cells in the brain that "wake up" these underactive regions.

Patient Experience: The patient is placed comfortably in a reclining chair and a coil is placed on top/side of the head. During the procedure, the patient will feel a burst of fast, light taps where the coil is placed. These bursts occur every 5–10 s and the entire procedure lasts 20–30 min. The procedure is repeated 5 days a week for 4–6 weeks totaling 20–30 sessions.

Side Effects: The most common side effect is pain or tingling at or near the treatment site. Other side effects include headache, dizziness, or light-headedness, extremely rare risk of seizure, or induction of mania.

Efficacy: TMS has been shown to have a response rate of 50% to 60% with one third of those achieving remission.

Vagus Nerve Stimulator

Background: It is typically reserved as a "last resort" for patients that have failed numerous other treatment modalities. The vagus nerve stimulator (VNS) obtained FDA approval for treatment-resistant depression in 2005.

How It works: A surgeon implants a battery-operated device under the left clavicle with a wire that is connected to the left vagus nerve. The device sends electrical impulses to the vagus nerve which stimulates the locus coeruleus and dorsal Raphe nucleus in the brain. The Raphe nucleus is thought to be linked to depression, and the locus coeruleus influences areas of the brain related to emotion. It is believed that the increased stimulation will improve depressive symptoms.

Patient Experience: The patient will be prepped just as they would for any general surgery that requires anesthesia. The procedure takes approximately 1–2 h. A small incision is made under the left chest where a pulse-producing device is implanted. Another small incision is made on the left side of the neck where the wire is connected to the vagus nerve. Recovery time from the procedure is minimal. Once implanted, the device will send an electric impulse that typically lasts for 30 s every 5 min. The patient will be able to feel the impulse, but it is usually not painful. The device can also be externally tuned using a magnet as subsequent follow-up visits.

Side Effects: Hoarseness, cough, and dyspnea are the most common side effects and usually present while the device is firing. There are also risks similar to those of general surgery including surgery site infection and adverse reactions to anesthesia.

Efficacy: The efficacy of VNS increases with time. In the original study comparing VNS to placebo, VNS did not show a clinically significant benefit at the 10 weeks versus placebo. However, at the 1-year mark, response rates for VNS were 46% with remission rates at 29%. While it appears that VNS does not appear as efficacious as other interventions, many of the people that receive VNS have already failed other modalities, including ECT. The patients undergoing VNS insertion typically have a more severe illness course [34].

Dysthymia

Dysthymia, also known as persistent depressive disorder, is a mood disorder sharing many similarities to MDD including hopelessness, anergia, and disruptions in cognition. It is typically milder in intensity compared to MDD but also longer in duration.

Diagnosing and Monitoring

Mnemonic: Two symptoms plus depressed mood for 2 years.

HE'S 2 SAD: **H**opelessness, **E**nergy loss, **S**elf-esteem is low, **2** years minimum, **S**leep increased or decreased, **A**ppetite is increased/decreased, **D**ecision-making is impaired [1].

DSM-5-TR

A persistent depressive disorder diagnoses require the person to have a depressed mood for the past 2 years, and the depressed mood must be present more days than not. It also requires two of the following symptoms in the presence of a depressed mood [2, p. 193]:

1. Poor appetite or overeating
2. Insomnia or hypersomnia
3. Low energy or fatigue
4. Low self-esteem
5. Poor concentration or difficulty making decisions
6. Feelings of hopelessness

The patient cannot be without symptoms for more than 6 months consecutively and it must interfere with daily life. The patient cannot have been diagnosed with a major depressive disorder or (hypo)manic episode. Finally, the condition is not better explained by a medical condition, drug/medication, or other mental illness that would better describe the symptoms [2].

Risk Factors: Genetic predisposition, first-degree relative with MDD, first-degree relative with dysthymic disorder, female gender.

Differential Diagnosis: Major depressive disorder, bipolar disorder, cyclothymic disorder, anxiety disorders, personality disorders, substance-induced disorders, and physical disorders similar to MDD.

Labs to Consider: Complete blood count (CBC), complete metabolic panel (CMP) thyroid functioning tests, B12 levels, vitamin D, and folate levels. Urine drug screen if warranted. If the patient reports snoring, excessive daytime sleepiness, or apnea, consider sleep study.

Treatment Options

There are no FDA-approved medications for persistent depressive disorder. Treatment modalities are similar to that of major depressive disorder. A combination of psychotherapy and pharmacology is the best approach. Cognitive behavioral analysis system of psychotherapy (CBASP) is a newer therapy specifically developed for managing chronic depression and may be beneficial in the treatment of PDD.

Seasonal Affective Disorder (SAD)

Major depressive disorder with seasonal pattern, formerly known as seasonal affective disorder, is a mood disorder characterized by depressive episodes or exacerbations recurring in late fall and winter, then alternating with euthymia beginning in the spring.

Diagnosing and Monitoring

DSM-5-TR

See page 2 for full Major Depressive Disorder Criteria.

Seasonal pattern modifier may be used if there is a relationship between a particular time of year (winter) and a depressive episode, the episode improves a certain time of year (spring), and it is recurrent for at least 2 years. See DSM-5-TR for full criteria and modifier.

Differential Diagnoses: Bipolar disorder, cyclothymic disorder, dysthymic disorder, premenstrual dysphoric disorder, chronic fatigue syndrome, hypothyroidism, and drug or alcohol abuse [35].

Risk Factors for SAD: Northern latitudes/living far from the equator, family history, female sex, diagnosis of depression or bipolar, and young age.

Labs to Consider: Complete blood count (CBC), complete metabolic panel (CMP) thyroid functioning tests, B12 levels, vitamin D, and folate levels. Urine drug screen if warranted. If the patient reports snoring, excessive daytime sleepiness, or apnea, consider sleep study.

Screening Scales

Seasonal Pattern Assessment Questionnaire (SPAQ): **It is a** 6-item instrument to assess how a subject's mood and behavior change over months and seasons. It is useful in initial assessment for suspected SAD.

PHQ-9: It is a 9-question, self-administered diagnostic tool that rates the severity of depression based on the last 2 weeks. It takes less than 3 min to complete and is the most popular depression screener. Using a cut-off value of 10, sensitivity and specificity is 85% and 85% [5].

Treatment

Non-pharmacologic Interventions

CBT-SAD: Cognitive behavioral therapy for the treatment of seasonal affective disorder as the name suggests is a variant of CBT specifically for those patients diagnosed with SAD. The therapy focuses on identifying negative thoughts and behaviors while replacing them with more positive ones [35].

Light Therapy: Using a light box with a minimum output of 10,000 lux of light, the patient is exposed to the light within the first hour of waking up in the morning for generally 20–30 min. The box is set up approximately 16–24 in. from the face. Exposure time can be titrated up to effect similar to titrating medications [35].

Pharmacologic Interventions

While all SSRIs seem to be beneficial for treating SAD, a 2022 review showed the three most promising medications for SAD are Zoloft, Prozac, and moclobemide. Given the side effect profile and dietary restrictions associated with moclobemide, Zoloft and Prozac are more highly recommended first-line medications. Wellbutrin is the only FDA-approved medication for SAD and is best served as a preventative approach, starting the medication in the fall prior to the patient becoming symptomatic.

Fluoxetine (Prozac)

Starting Dose: 20 mg PO daily. 10 mg PO daily can be used in elderly.

Titration: Increase by 20 mg PO daily after 1 week. Wait for 4–6 weeks for the response when initializing therapy.

Max Dose: 80 mg PO daily.

FDA Approval: MDD (8 and older), OCD (7 and older), PMDD, bulimia, panic disorder.

Common Side Effects: GI upset, sexual dysfunction, insomnia, anxiety, agitation, headache, dizziness, sweating, bruising, and nausea, which should improve in 3–5 days.

Rare: *Seizures, hyponatremia, induction of mania, Serotonin Syndrome, bleeding, SIADH, and activation of suicidal ideation in those under 24.*

Monitoring: PHQ-9, ECG if QT prolongation. Height and weight on children.

Pearl: No need to taper off medication when discontinuing due to long half-life.

Contraindications: Taking MAO-I, thioridazine, pimozide, and known hypersensitivity to fluoxetine.

Black Box Warning: Use may increase suicidal thoughts in children, adolescents, and young adults (24 and younger) [13].

Sertraline (Zoloft)

Starting Dose: 50 mg PO daily. 25 mg PO daily in elderly.

Titration: Increase by 25–50 mg PO daily every week. Wait for 4–6 weeks for the response when initializing therapy.

Max Dose: 200 mg PO daily.

FDA Approval: Major depressive disorder (MDD), obsessive compulsive disorder (OCD), panic disorder, posttraumatic stress disorder (PTSD), premenstrual dysphoric disorder (PMDD), social anxiety disorder.

Common Side Effects: GI upset, sexual dysfunction, agitation, headache, insomnia, sedation, sweating, bruising, and nausea, which should improve in 3–5 days.

Rare: *Seizures, hyponatremia, induction of mania, hypotension, Serotonin Syndrome, bleeding, SIADH, and activation of suicidal ideation in those under 24.*

Monitoring: PHQ-9.

Contraindications: Taking MAO-I, pimozide, and known hypersensitivity to Sertraline. Avoid in untreated angle-closure glaucoma.

Black Box Warning: Use may increase suicidal thoughts in children, adolescents, and young adults (24 and younger) [16].

Bupropion XL (Wellbutrin XL): Norepinephrine and Dopamine Reuptake Inhibitor (NDRI)

Starting Dose: 150 mg PO daily.

Titration: Increase by 150 mg PO daily. Wait for 4–6 weeks for the response when initializing therapy.

Max Dose: 450 mg PO daily.

FDA Approval: MDD, seasonal affective disorder, nicotine addiction (standard release).

Common Side Effects: Dry mouth, constipation, GI upset, insomnia, dizziness, headache, agitation, anxiety, tremor, sweating, weight loss, anorexia, myalgia, tinnitus, rash, and hypertension.

Rare: *Seizures, Stevens-Johnson syndrome has been reported, induction of mania, and activation of suicidal ideation in those under 24.*

Monitoring: PHQ-9 and blood pressure.

PEARL: XL only requires once a day dosing, making it the preferred preparation. It can be given with other antidepressants to help with sexual side effects.

Contraindicated: Patients with current or prior diagnosis of bulimia or anorexia nervosa. Patients with a history of seizures. If a patient is abruptly quitting alcohol, sedative use, or anticonvulsant medication. If a patient has had a recent head injury or has a nervous system tumor. Taking a MAO-I or Thioridazine [22].

Postpartum Depression

Postpartum depression (PPD), now known as major depressive disorder with peripartum onset, is a serious mood disorder occurring in women shortly after delivering a child. It is estimated that up to 50% of peripartum onset actually begins prior to delivery. The DSM-V requires the onset be within 4 weeks of delivery. However, others define it broadly, within the first year of delivery.

Diagnosing and Monitoring

DSM-TR-5

See page 2 for full Major Depressive Disorder Criteria.

Use the peripartum onset specifier of MDD episode present during pregnancy or up to 4 weeks after birth.

Differential Diagnoses: "Baby blues," thyroid dysfunction, postpartum psychosis.

Risk Factors for Postpartum Depression: Depression during pregnancy, history of depression perinatal or postpartum, stressful life event prior to delivery, high risk pregnancy, spousal abuse during pregnancy, family history of PPD, and smoking during pregnancy.

Screening Scales

Edinburgh Postnatal Depression Scale (EPDS)— It is 10-question, self-administered questionnaire that only takes a few minutes to complete. A cutoff score equal to or greater than 13 is required to determine if patients are at risk for developing PPD.

PHQ-9—It is a 9-question, self-administered diagnostic tool that rates the severity of depression based on the last 2 weeks. It takes less than 3 min to complete and is the most popular depression screener. Using a cut-off value of 10, sensitivity and specificity is 85% and 85%.

HAM-D—It consists of 21 questions with only 17 being scored for severity of depression. It is clinician administered and more in depth while also being more time consuming than PHQ-9. It takes about 15 min to complete. Sensitivity and specificity values will vary based on the specific cutoff scores chosen for the HAM-D and the population being tested.

****It is important to use the same scale consistently.* ***

Treatment

Treatment options are dependent on the severity of the illness. To determine severity, screening tools can be helpful. Mild severity is a score of 5–9 on the PHQ-9 or less than 11 on the EPDS. Moderate severity is a score of 10–19 on the PHQ-9 or 12–15 on the EPDS [36].

Mild to Moderate PPD

For mild to moderate PPD that is the first occurrence of depression, first-line treatment is psychotherapy. If there is failure of the initial psychotherapy, it is recommended to try a different type of psychotherapy before starting medications. If there is a history of depressive episodes prior to PPD, it would be prudent to start with pharmacotherapy. Pharmacotherapy can be used if psychotherapy is not available, patient preference for medication, or there is a failure of two distinct types of psychotherapy [36].

Non-pharmacologic Interventions

Cognitive Behavioral Therapy (CBT): It is a type of therapy that focuses on changing one's thoughts and behaviors to improve mood and functioning. It has been adapted for postpartum depression.

Interpersonal Therapy (IPT): It is a type of therapy that focuses on interpersonal relationships and social interactions that can have an impact on your mental health. It has also been adapted to be used in PPD.

Behavioral Activation Therapy: It is a type of therapy that teaches the patient increase adaptive and rewarding activities, builds problem-solving skills, and decreases withdrawal and avoidance behaviors that may exacerbate depression. Behavioral activation therapy has been shown to be as efficacious as antidepressants in unipolar depressed patients.

Severe PPD

A severe score for PPD is 20 and above for the PHQ-9 and 16 and above on the EPDS. Severe illness can also include patients with suicidal/homicidal ideations, catatonia, delusions/hallucinations, or grossly impaired motor function. Severely ill patients should not be left alone with their infant, and hospitalization should be considered if the patient is a threat to themselves or others. Pharmacotherapy is a preferred modality of treatment for severe PPD but in combination with psychotherapy may prove more beneficial.

If the patient has been on successful antidepressant therapy prior, it is recommended to restart the same medication as it is generally accepted that benefit outweighs the risk. If the patient was on a medication during pregnancy, it is preferable to continue or restart the same medication. If patient is medication naïve, Paxil and Zoloft are the preferable choice due to low bioavailability in breast milk.

For those that prefer rapid onset of relief, intravenous brexanolone can be considered. Brexanolone is a neuroactive steroid that is administered intravenously over a 60-h infusion. It must be administered at a certified healthcare facility through the Risk Evaluation and Mitigation Strategy (REMS). Close monitoring of vitals and level of consciousness is needed throughout the administration process. Brexanolone can provide benefit in as little as 24 h. In August of 2023, the FDA approved the first oral treatment for PPD, zuranolone. Zuranolone is given by mouth daily for 14 days and may be preferable to an IV infusion. As of the time of this publication, zuranolone has not been placed on the market so there is no information on dosing.

Electroconvulsive therapy (ECT) is a treatment option in severe cases and for patients wanting a rapid response. ECT is done in the hospital under general anesthesia. The anesthesiologist will sedate the patient, and then the doctor performing the procedure will use electrodes to introduce electrical stimuli to a specific area of the brain that will in turn elicit a seizure that lasts approximately 30–60 s. The patient wakes up within 5–10 min and stays in recovery for approximately 30 min. ECT is done 2–3 times a week for a total of 6–12 sessions [36].

Medications

Paroxetine (Paxil)

Starting Dose:

Immediate Release: 20 mg PO daily. 10 mg PO daily can be used in elderly.

Controlled Release: 25 mg PO daily.

Titration:

Immediate Release: Increase by 10 mg PO daily, after 1 week. Wait for 4–6 weeks for the response when initializing therapy.

Controlled Release: 12.5 mg po daily, after 1 week. Wait for 4–6 weeks for the response when initializing therapy.

Max Dose:

Immediate Release: 50 mg PO daily.

Controlled Release: 62.5 mg po daily.

FDA Approval: MDD, OCD, panic disorder, SAD, PTSD, GAD, PMDD

Common Side Effects: GI upset, sexual dysfunction, agitation, headache, sedation, dizziness, tremor, bruising, weight gain, nausea (better in 3–5 days).

Rare: *Seizures, hyponatremia, induction of mania, serotonin syndrome, bleeding, SIADH, and activation of suicidal ideation in those under 24.*

Monitoring: PHQ-9.

Pearl: There is a need to wean over several months for those who cannot tolerate withdrawal effects.

Contraindications: Taking MAO-I, pimozide, and known hypersensitivity to paroxetine.

Black Box Warning: Use may increase suicidal thoughts in children, adolescents, and young adults (24 and younger) ([14, 15].

*****Beers List for drugs to avoid in the elderly*****

Sertraline (Zoloft)

Starting Dose: 50 mg PO daily. 25 mg PO daily in elderly.

Titration: Increase by 25–50 mg PO daily every week. Wait for 4–6 weeks for the response when initializing therapy.

Max Dose: 200 mg PO daily.

FDA Approval: Major depressive disorder (MDD), obsessive compulsive disorder (OCD), panic disorder, posttraumatic stress disorder (PTSD), premenstrual dysphoric disorder (PMDD), social anxiety disorder.

Common Side Effects: GI upset, sexual dysfunction, agitation, headache, insomnia, sedation, sweating, bruising, and nausea (better in 3–5 days).

Rare: *Seizures, hyponatremia, induction of mania, hypotension, serotonin syndrome, and activation of suicidal ideation in those under 24*. Bleeding and SIADH.

Monitoring: PHQ-9.

Contraindications: Taking MAO-I, thioridazine, pimozide, or tamoxifen.

Black Box Warning: Use may increase suicidal thoughts in children, adolescents, and young adults (24 and younger) [16].

Premenstrual Dysphoric Disorder

Premenstrual dysphoric disorder (PMDD) is a mood disorder causing physical, cognitive, and affective symptoms in women during their menstrual cycle. Onset of symptoms start at the beginning of the late luteal phase and typically resolve at the onset of menses.

Diagnosing and Monitoring

DSM-5-TR

For a PMDD diagnosis, patients must have symptom onset the week prior to menses, improve after onset, and then be asymptomatic (or close) in the next few weeks. One or more bolded symptoms must be present and at least one other symptoms for a total of five ([2], p. 197):

1. **Mood lability**
2. **Irritability or anger or increased interpersonal conflicts**

3. **Depressed mood, feelings of hopelessness, or self-deprecating thoughts**
4. **Anxiety, tension, or feeling on edge**
5. Decreased interest
6. Difficulty concentration
7. Decreased energy
8. Significant appetite changes
9. Sleep disturbances: too much/too little
10. Feeling overwhelmed or out of control
11. Breast tenderness or swelling, joint or muscle pain, a sensation of "bloating," or weight gain

For the diagnosis to be made, it has to have a significant impact on daily life. It cannot be an exacerbation of another mood disorder, or be better explained by a medical cause or drug. Symptoms should be tracked with a prospective dialing rating scale and have two positive months before confirming the diagnoses [2].

Differential Diagnoses: Mood disorders (bipolar, MDD), anxiety disorders, menopausal transition, thyroid disorders, substance abuse, and other medical conditions (e.g., chronic fatigue syndrome, migraines, mastalgia).

Risk Factors for PMDD: Posttraumatic events, cigarette smoking, obesity, and possibly genetics.

Labs to Consider: Thyroid panel to rule out hypo/hyperthyroidism, complete blood count, and follicle stimulating hormone (FSH) to rule out perimenopause. Hormonal patterns in patients with PMDD are typically normal, hormonal shift is not the cause, but it is the sensitivity to those shifts.

Screening Scales

Premenstrual Symptom Screening Tool (PSST): **It is** a questionnaire created to aid in the diagnosis of PMDD. The PSST consists of 19 questions that assess the severity of PMS/PMDD symptoms and how they interfere with daily activities and relationships.

Daily Record of Severity of Problems (DRSP): Prospective symptom monitoring is the gold standard diagnosis for PMDD, and the DRSP is a validated tool to help assist with the diagnosis. It is a scale that consists of 24 items, out of which 21 are grouped into 11 distinct symptoms and 3 functional impairment items. Each item is rated on a scale from 1 to 6 with 1 being not at all and 6 being extreme.

Treatment

There is a litany of research for the treatment of PMDD ranging from SSRIs dosing during the luteal phase to hysterectomy with bilateral salpingectomy/oophorectomy (BSO). The treatments with the most robust research are the use of SSRIs, combined oral contraceptives, and psychotherapy for those with mild symptoms that do not want to take medications [37].

Non-pharmacologic Interventions

Cognitive Behavioral Therapy (CBT): It is a type of therapy that focuses on changing one's thoughts and behaviors to improve mood and functioning. It has been adapted for premenstrual dysphoric disorder.

Mindfulness-Based Cognitive Behavioral Therapy (MCBT): It is a type of therapy that combines traditional CBT with mindfulness medication practices. Originally developed to prevent MDD relapse, MCBT focuses on being in the present moment and trying to achieve a non-judgmental attitude called "mindfulness."

Medications

The most studied medications for PMDD are Zoloft, Lexapro, Paxil, Prozac, and Effexor. Research has shown similar efficacy between continuous treatment and luteal phase dosing with continuous treatment slightly outperforming. Of note, studies have shown no significant discontinuation symptoms in the intermittent dosing of Zoloft, so treatment strategy should be patient preference. The following are suggested doses for luteal phase dosing, see antidepressant section for more detailed prescribing notes. Bold medications are FDA approved.

Escitalopram (Lexapro)	10–20 mg daily
Fluoxetine (Sarafem)	10–20 mg daily
Paroxetine (Paxil)	10–20 mg daily
Paroxetine CR (Paxil CR)	12.5–25 mg daily
Sertraline (Zoloft)	50–100 mg daily
Venlafaxine (Effexor XR)	75–112.5 mg daily

Combined oral contraceptives (COC) have also showed promise for treatment of PMDD with drospirenone/ethinyl estradiol (Yaz) and drospirenone/ethinyl estradiol/levomefolate (Beyaz) being the only FDA-approved COC medications for PMDD. Prescribing COC is outside of the scope of this book, and prescribing should be done under the guidance of an OB/GYN [37].

References

1. Caplan J, Stern T. Mnemonics in a mnutshell: 32 aids to psychiatric diagnosis. Curr Psychiatr Ther. 2008;7(10):27–33.
2. American Psychiatric Association. Depressive disorders. In: Diagnostic and statistical manual of mental disorders (5th-TR). Washington, DC: American Psychiatric Association; 2022.
3. Major Depressive Disorder | Johns Hopkins Psychiatry Guide; 2022, May 8. https://www.hopkinsguides.com/hopkins/view/Johns_Hopkins_Psychiatry_Guide/787049/all/Major_Depressive_Disorder
4. Maurer DM. Screening for depression. AAFP; 2012, January 15. https://www.aafp.org/pubs/afp/issues/2012/0115/p139.html.
5. Negeri, Z., Levis, B., Sun, Y., He, C., Krishnan, A., Wu, Y., Bhandari, P. M., Neupane, D., Brehaut, E., Benedetti, A., & Thombs, B. D. (2021). Accuracy of the Patient Health Questionnaire-9 for screening to detect major depression: updated systematic review and individual participant data meta-analysis BMJ, n2183. doi: https://doi.org/10.1136/bmj.n2183.
6. Timmerby N, Andersen JH, Søndergaard S, Østergaard SD, Bech P. A systematic review of the clinimetric properties of the 6-item version of the Hamilton Depression Rating Scale (HAM-D6). Psychother Psychosom. 2017;86(3):141–9. https://doi.org/10.1159/000457131. Epub 2017 May 11.

7. Quick Inventory of Depressive Symptomatology (QIDS) | NP Psych Navigator; n.d. https://www.nppsychnavigator.com/Clinical-Tools/Psychiatric-Scales/Quick-Inventory-of-Depressive-Symptomatology-(QIDS).
8. Cuijpers P, Karyotaki E, Ciharova M, Miguel C, Noma H, Furukawa TA. The effects of psychotherapies for depression on response, remission, reliable change, and deterioration: a meta-analysis. Acta Psychiatr Scand. 2021;144(3):288–99. https://doi.org/10.1111/acps.13335. Epub 2021 Jul 4.
9. Gaynes BN, Rush AJ, Wisniewski SR, Spencer D, Fava M, Trivedi MH. The STAR*D study: treating depression in the real world. Cleveland Clin J Med. 2008;75(1):57–8. https://www.ccjm.org/content/ccjom/75/1/57.full.pdf
10. Homepage | WILD 5. (n.d.). https://wild5wellnessprogram.com/.
11. AbbVie. Celexa: highlights of prescribing information; 2023. https://www.rxabbvie.com/pdf/celexa_pi.pdf.
12. Forest Pharmaceuticals, Inc. Lexapro: Highlights of prescribing information; 2009. https://www.accessdata.fda.gov/drugsatfda_docs/label/2009/021323s030s031,021365s021s022lbl.pdf.
13. Eli Lilly and Company. Prozac: highlights of prescribing information; 1987. https://pi.lilly.com/us/prozac.pdf.
14. GlaxoSmithKline. Paxil: prescribing information; 2008. https://www.accessdata.fda.gov/drugsatfda_docs/label/2008/020031s060,020936s037,020710s024lbl.pdf.
15. GlaxoSmithKline. Paxil CR: prescribing information; 2014. https://www.accessdata.fda.gov/drugsatfda_docs/label/2014/020936s049lbl.pdf.
16. Pfizer. Zoloft: highlights of prescribing information; 2021. https://labeling.pfizer.com/ShowLabeling.aspx?id=517.
17. AbbVie. Viibryd: highlights of prescribing information; 2023. https://www.rxabbvie.com/pdf/viibryd_pi.pdf.
18. Takeda Pharmaceuticals. Trintellix: highlights of prescribing information; 2023. https://www.accessdata.fda.gov/drugsatfda_docs/label/2021/204447s021s022lbl.pdf.
19. Pfizer. Pristiq: highlights of prescribing information; 2023. https://labeling.pfizer.com/showlabeling.aspx?id=497.
20. Eli Lilly and Company. Cymbalta: highlights of prescribing information; 2023. https://pi.lilly.com/us/cymbalta-pi.pdf.
21. Viatris Specialty LLC. Effexor XR: Highlights of Prescribing Information; 2023. https://www.accessdata.fda.gov/drugsatfda_docs/label/2023/020699s118lbl.pdf.
22. GlaxoSmithKline. Wellbutrin XL: prescribing information; 2009. https://www.accessdata.fda.gov/drugsatfda_docs/label/2009/021515s023s024lbl.pdf.
23. Axsome Therapeutics Inc. Auvelity: highlights of prescribing information; 2022. https://www.axsome.com/auvelity-prescribing-information.pdf.

24. Organon USA Inc. Remeron: prescribing information; 2007. https://www.accessdata.fda.gov/drugsatfda_docs/label/2007/020415s019,021208s010lbl.pdf.
25. Pragma Pharmaceuticals, Inc. Desyrel: highlights of prescribing information; 2017. https://www.accessdata.fda.gov/drugsatfda_docs/label/2017/018207s032lbl.pdf.
26. Otsuka American Pharmaceutical, Inc. Abilify: highlights of prescribing information; 2022. https://www.otsuka-us.com/sites/g/files/qhldwo7626/files/media/static/Abilify-PI.pdf.
27. Otsuka Pharmaceutical Co. Rexulti: highlights of prescribing information; 2023. https://otsuka-us.com/sites/g/files/qhldwo7626/files/media/static/Rexulti-PI.pdf.
28. Forest Laboratories Holdings Ltd. Vraylar: highlights of prescribing information; 2022. https://www.rxabbvie.com/pdf/vraylar_pi.pdf.
29. Eli Lilly and Company. Symbyax: highlights of prescribing information; 2023. https://pi.lilly.com/us/symbyax-pi.pdf.
30. AstraZeneca Pharmaceuticals LP. Seroquel XR: highlights of prescribing information; 2009. https://www.accessdata.fda.gov/drugsatfda_docs/label/2009/022047s011s016s017s019s022lbl.pdf.
31. Mughal S. Postpartum depression. StatPearls - NCBI Bookshelf; 2022, October 7. https://www.ncbi.nlm.nih.gov/books/NBK519070/.
32. Park MJ, Kim H, Kim YH, Yook V, Chung IW, Lee SM, Jeon HJ. Recent updates on electro-convulsive therapy in patients with depression. Psychiatr Investig. 2021;18(1):1–10. https://doi.org/10.30773/pi.2020.0350.
33. Popova V, Daly E, Trivedi MH, Cooper K, Lane R, Lim P, Mazzucco C, Hough D, Thase ME, Shelton RC, Molero P, Vieta E, Bajbouj M, Manji HK, Drevets WC, Singh J. Efficacy and safety of flexibly dosed Esketamine nasal Spray combined with a newly initiated oral antidepressant in Treatment-Resistant Depression: a randomized Double-Blind Active-Controlled study. Am J Psychiatr. 2019;176(6):428–38. https://doi.org/10.1176/appi.ajp.2019.19020172.
34. O'Reardon JP. Vagus Nerve stimulation (VNS) and treatment of depression: to the brainstem and beyond. PubMed Central (PMC); n.d. https://www.ncbi.nlm.nih.gov/pmc/articles/PMC2990624/.
35. Kurlansik SL, Ibay AD. Seasonal affective disorder. AAFP; 2012, December 1. https://www.aafp.org/pubs/afp/issues/2012/1201/p1037.html.
36. Postpartum Depression: Action Towards Causes and Treatment (PACT) Consortium. Heterogeneity of postpartum depression: a latent class analysis. Lancet Psychiatry. 2015;2(1):59–67. https://doi.org/10.1016/S2215-0366(14)00055-8. Epub 2015 Jan 8.

37. Carlini SV, di Scalea LT, McNally ST, Lester J, Deligiannidis KM. Management of premenstrual dysphoric disorder: a scoping review. Int J Womens Health. 2022;14:1783–801. https://doi.org/10.2147/IJWH.S297062.

Anxiety Disorders

2

Contents

B. Floyd, T. Kane, *The Clinician's Guide to Common Psychiatric Disorders*, https://doi.org/10.1007/978-3-031-67958-2_2

Generalized Anxiety Disorder

Generalized anxiety disorder (GAD) is a mental health condition that is hallmarked by persistent and excessive worry about everyday life events. The worry is typically disproportionate to the actual circumstances. GAD is often accompanied by somatic symptoms such as fatigue, muscle tension, nausea, and sweating.

Diagnosing and Monitoring

Mnemonic: Worry or anxiety plus 3 symptoms lasting a minimum of 6 months.

WATCHERS: **W**orry/**A**nxiety, plus: **T**ension in muscles, **C**oncentration difficulty, **H**yperarousal/irritable, **E**nergy loss, **R**estlessness, **S**leep disturbances [1].

DSM-5-TR

To have a diagnosis of generalized anxiety disorder according to the DSM-5-TR, the patient must have excessive worrying or anxiety for at least 6 months. The anxiety should be present at most than not and adversely affect daily functioning. The anxiety is difficult to control and they must have three of the following six symptoms [2, p. 250]:

1. Feeling on edge or being restless
2. Decreased energy reserves/Easily Fatigued
3. Difficulty concentrating
4. Irritability
5. Muscle tension
6. Sleep disturbances

The anxiety will cause significant dysfunction in an area of life such as work or social settings. Finally, the anxiety is not the result of a physiological process and drug or better explained by another mental illness.

Differential Diagnoses: Adrenal crisis, alcoholism, amphetamine-related psychiatric disorders, anorexia, A fib, caffeine-related disorders, cannabis-related disorders, delirium, depression, dysthymia, hallucinogen use, insomnia, OCD, phobic disorders, PDD, schizoaffective, schizophrenia, stimulant use, thyroiditis, T1DM, and unstable angina [3].

Risk Factors for GAD: Female sex, chronic illness, substance abuse, family history, and stressful life event [4].

Labs to Consider: CBC, CMP, TSH, urinalysis, electrocardiogram (in patients over 40 with chest pain or palpitations), and urine toxicology. It is extremely important to rule out any other medical causes.

Screening Scales

Generalized Anxiety Disorder 7 (GAD-7): It is a self-reported questionnaire for screening and severity of each symptom. It consists of 7 items, which measure severity of various symptoms of GAD. It is the most popular GAD screening tool. It has a sensitivity and specificity of 89% and 82% [5].

Hamilton Anxiety Rating Scale (HAM-A): It is a clinician-rated screening tool with a total of 14 questions. It is more in depth than GAD-7 and relies on clinician expertise [6].

Beck Anxiety Inventory (BAI): It is a 21-question multiple-choice self-report inventory that is used for measuring the severity of anxiety in adolescents and adults ages 17 and older.

****The scale used is not as important as using the same scale consistently.* ***

Treatment

Cognitive behavioral therapy (CBT) has a response rate that is approximately 50% when treating generalized anxiety disorder.

Studies also show that the response is sustained for months, even after terminating the therapy. Pharmacological interventions with SSRIs have a similar response rate at approximately 60%. Combination of CBT and pharmacotherapy is generally thought to be the most efficacious option. While other therapy options are available such as stress management and supportive counseling, CBT has the most data on efficacy in treating GAD. First-line treatment is a personal choice with some patient opting for medications, while others prefer trying therapy first. Both are valid approaches [7].

Non-pharmacologic Interventions

Cognitive Behavioral Therapy (CBT): It is a type of therapy that focuses on changing one's thoughts and behaviors to improve mood and functioning. It is a short-term, collaborative, goal-oriented therapy where the therapist helps the client identify negative thought patterns and behaviors, and they develop ways to reconceptualize these thoughts and behaviors into something more positive.

Treatment Recommendations: General Anxiety Disorder

First-Line Treatment: Start Selective Serotonin Reuptake Inhibitor

- If improvement is seen after 4–6 weeks, maximize dose.
- If there is no improvement after 4–6 weeks, switch SSRI.
- If partial response and dose is maximized, add Buspar.

  Second-Line Treatment: Attempt Second SSRI

- If improvement is seen after 4–6 weeks, maximize dose.
- If there is no improvement after 4–6 weeks, change class to SNRI.
- If partial response and dose is maximized, add Buspar or hydroxyzine.

Third-Line Treatment: Start SNRI

- If improvement is seen after 4–6 weeks, maximize dose.
- If there is no improvement, see off-label treatment resistant and refer to psychiatric specialist.
- If partial response and dose is maximized, add Buspar or hydroxyzine.

First-Line Medications: Generalized Anxiety Disorder

Duloxetine (Cymbalta)

Starting Dose: 40 mg PO daily.

Titration: Increase by 20 mg PO daily during first titration. Wait for 4–6 weeks for the response when initializing therapy. Then it may be increased by 30 mg PO daily.

Max Dose: 120 mg PO daily.

FDA Approval: MDD, diabetic peripheral neuropathy, fibromyalgia, GAD, chronic musculoskeletal pain.

Common Side Effects: INCREASED blood pressure, GI upset, sexual dysfunction, insomnia, agitation, sedation, dizziness, urinary retention, headache, and nausea, which should improve in 3–5 days.

Rare: *Seizures, hyponatremia, induction of mania, and activation of suicidal ideation in those under 24.*

Monitoring: PHQ-9, blood pressure at each visit.

PEARL: Patient may get benefit of pain reduction on 30 mg dose. This medication should be avoided for patients with hepatic insufficiency.

Contraindications: Angle-closure glaucoma, substantial alcohol use, taking a MAO-I, taking thioridazine.

Black Box Warning: Use may increase suicidal thoughts in children, adolescents, and young adults (24 and younger) [8]).

Escitalopram (Lexapro)

Starting Dose: 10 mg PO daily. 5 mg PO daily can be used in elderly.

Titration: Increase by 5–10 mg PO daily every week. Wait for 4–6 weeks for the response when initializing therapy.

Max Dose: 20 mg PO daily.

FDA Approval: MDD (12 and up) and generalized anxiety disorder (GAD).

Common Side Effects: *Fatigue, GI upset, sexual dysfunction, agitation, headache, and nausea, which should improve in 3–5 days.

Rare: *Seizures, hyponatremia, induction of mania, and activation of suicidal ideation in those under 24.*

Monitoring: PHQ-9, ECG if QT prolongation, and height and weight on children.

Pearl: Lexapro has the best side effect profile of all SSRIs.

Contraindications: Taking a MAO-I or pimozide.

Black Box Warning: Use may increase suicidal thoughts in children, adolescents, and young adults (24 and younger) [9].

Paroxetine (Paxil)

Starting Dose: Immediate Release: 20 mg PO daily. 10 mg PO daily can be used in elderly.

Controlled Release: 25 mg PO daily.

Titration: Immediate Release: Increase by 10 mg PO daily every week.

Controlled Release: 12.5 mg po daily. Wait for 4–6 weeks for the response when initializing therapy.

Max Dose: Immediate Release: 50 mg PO daily.

Controlled Release: 62.5 mg po daily.

FDA Approval: MDD, OCD, panic disorder, SAD, PTSD, GAD, PMDD.

Common Side Effects: GI upset, sexual dysfunction, agitation, headache, and nausea, which should improve in 3–5 days.

Rare: *Seizures, hyponatremia, induction of mania, and activation of suicidal ideation in those under 24.*

Monitoring: PHQ-9.

Pearl: There is a need to wean over several months for those who cannot tolerate withdrawal effects.

Contraindications: Taking MAO-I, thioridazine, pimozide, or tamoxifen.

Black Box Warning: Use may increase suicidal thoughts in children, adolescents, and young adults (24 and younger) [10, 11].

*****Beers List for drugs to avoid in the elderly*****

Venlafaxine XR (Effexor XR)

Starting Dose: 37.5 mg PO daily.

Titration: Increase by 37.5 mg PO daily in 1 week. Then, titrate by 75 mg PO daily. Wait for 4–6 weeks (on 75 mg dose) for the response when initializing therapy.

Max Dose: 375 mg PO daily.

FDA Approval: Depression, GAD, SAD, panic disorder, separation anxiety disorder.

Common Side Effects: INCREASED blood pressure, GI upset, sexual dysfunction, insomnia, agitation, anxiety, sweating, headache, and nausea, which should improve in 3–5 days.

Rare: *Seizures, hyponatremia, induction of mania, and activation of suicidal ideation in those under 24.*

Monitoring: PHQ-9, blood pressure at each visit.

Pearls: Higher doses are associated with more side effects. Immediate release forms are available but are more prone to discontinuation syndrome. Effexor can be difficult to wean. Alternative strategies may need to be used and length of titration may take months. Patients commonly report "brain zaps" while discontinuing or even missing a dose.

Contraindications: Uncontrolled angle-closure glaucoma or taking a MAO-I.

Black Box Warning: Use may increase suicidal thoughts in children, adolescents, and young adults (24 and younger) [12].

*** All other SSRIs and antidepressants are considered off label but are equally efficacious. ***

Second-Line Medications

Buspirone (Buspar)

Starting Dose: 5 mg PO daily.

Titration: Increase to 5 mg PO BID after 5–7 days. BID dosing is usually the easiest.

Max Dose: 60 mg/day.

FDA Approval: Management of anxiety disorders.

Common Side Effects: Dizziness, nervousness, sedation, GI issues, headache, agitation.

Rare: *Cardiac symptoms.*

Monitoring: GAD-7.

Pearl: It should be taken every day as scheduled for best efficacy and should NOT be used as needed.

Contraindication: Taking a MAO-I [13].

Hydroxyzine (Vistaril)

Starting Dose: 25 mg PO every 6 h.

Titration: It may go up in 25 mg increments q 6 h.

Max Dose: 100 mg 4 times daily.

FDA Approval: Anxiety and tension associated with psychoneurosis, pruritis due to allergic condition, histamine-mediated pruritis, premedication sedation, acute hysteria, anxiety withdrawal symptoms in alcoholics, nausea, and vomiting.

Off-Label: Insomnia.

Common Side Effects: Dry mouth, drowsiness, GI issues, headache, agitation.

Monitoring: GAD-7.

Pearl: Take at first sign of anxiety.

Contraindication: Early-stage pregnancy, patients with prolonged QT interval, and known hypersensitivity to hydroxyzine [14].

*****Beers List for drugs to avoid in the elderly*****

Benzodiazepines

Benzodiazepines are considered second-line treatments. They should be used at the lowest effective dose for the shortest amount of time possible.

*****Beers List for drugs to avoid in the elderly*****

Alprazolam (Xanax)

Starting Dose: 0.25 mg PO (Daily to TID) PRN.

Titration: 0.25 mg to 0.5 mg PO (Daily to TID).

Max Dose: 3 mg/day.

FDA Approval: Generalized anxiety disorder and panic disorder.

Off-Label Disorders: Other anxiety disorders, anxiety associated with depression, IBS, acute mania, acute psychosis, and catatonia.

Common Side Effects: Sedation, fatigue, depression, dizziness, ataxia, slurred speech, weakness, forgetfulness, confusion, hyperexcitability, nervousness, dry mouth, mania, hypotension, *respiratory depression*.

Rare: *Hepatic dysfunction, renal dysfunction, blood dyscrasias.*

Monitoring: GAD-7.

Pearl: Withdrawal can occur with prolonged use, and patient will need expert guidance on discontinuing medication. DO NOT MIX WITH ALCOHOL.

Contraindicated: Angle-closure glaucoma or with concomitant azole use [15, 16].

Panic Disorder

Panic attacks are intense bouts of fear, anxiety, or discomfort that typically last a short period of time. A patient having one panic attack does not necessarily mean he or she has a panic disorder. Panic disorder is hallmarked by maladaptive behaviors related to the panic attacks either by way of avoidance or persistent worry that interrupts everyday life.

Is It Panic or Anxiety?

	Anxiety	Panic
Cause	Usually caused by something (i.e., stressful job, new situation)	"Out of the Blue"
Timing	Builds gradually culminating in attack	Almost immediately. No preceding factors
Severity	Mild, moderate, or severe	Severe and debilitating
Effect	Can lead to further anxiety about the cause	Can create fear of having another attack. Maladaptive behaviors

Diagnosing and Monitoring

Mnemonic: Abrupt surge of intense fear that peaks within minutes accompanied by four or more symptoms.

STUDENTS FEAR 3 Cs: **S**weating, **T**rembling, **U**nsteadiness, **D**epersonalization/**D**erealization, **E**xcessive heart rate, **N**ausea, **T**ingling, and **S**hortness of breath. **Fear** = (1) dying and (2) losing control or going crazy. **Cs**: **C**hest pain, **C**hills, and **C**hoking [1].

DSM-5-TR

According to the DSM-5-TR, a panic attack is "an abrupt surge of intense fear of intense discomfort." It peaks quickly, usually within a few minutes, and at least four of the following symptoms are present [2, p. 235]:

1. Palpitations, pounding heart, or accelerated heart rate
2. Sweating
3. Trembling or shaking
4. Sensations of shortness of breath or smothering
5. Feelings of choking
6. Chest pain or discomfort
7. Nausea or abdominal distress
8. Feeling dizzy, unsteady, light-headed, or faint
9. Chills or heat sensations
10. Paresthesias (numbness or tingling sensations)
11. Derealizations (feelings of unreality) or depersonalization (being detached from oneself)
12. Fear of losing control or "going crazy"
13. Fear of dying

Having a panic attack does not mean the patient has panic disorder. In order for the diagnosis to be made, additional criteria are needed. After a panic attack, there has to be a 1 month period where the patient has persistent concern or worry about additional panic attacks or has maladaptive changes in behavior trying to avoid the panic attacks. Again, this cannot be the result of a physiological process and drug or better explained by another mental illness.

Differential Diagnosis: Hyperthyroidism, hyperparathyroidism, pheochromocytomas, vestibular dysfunction, seizure disorder, cardiac arrhythmias, CNS stimulant use, other anxious disorders, general medical disorder [17].

Screening Scales

The Panic Disorder Severity Scale (PDSS): It is a self-reported scale that measures the severity of panic attacks and panic disorder symptoms. It is designed for ages 13 and up.

The Severity Measure for Panic Disorder—Adult: It is a 10-item measure that assesses the severity of symptoms of panic disorder in individuals age 18 and older once they have received a diagnosis of panic disorder.

Panic Disorder Screener (PADIS): The first item is rated on a 5-point Likert scale scored 0–4, while the remaining items are rated on a 4-point Likert scale score 0–3. Severity scores are obtained by summing responses to all items, with scores ranging from 0 to 13 [18].

Treatment

Treatment depends on severity of symptoms, frequency of symptoms, and patient preference. A patient with mild to moderate intermittent symptoms that do not dramatically impact quality of life may opt to forego treatment and use a watchful waiting approach. Those with more serious and debilitating symptoms should be treated with CBT or medication with a combination approach offering the best efficacy. Those with comorbid psychiatric illnesses will usually require medication.

First-Line Medications: Panic Disorder

Fluoxetine (Prozac)

Starting Dose: 20 mg PO daily. 10 mg PO daily can be used in elderly.

Titration: Increase by 20 mg PO daily every week. Wait for 4–6 weeks for the response when initializing therapy.

Max Dose: 80 mg PO daily.

FDA Approval: MDD (8 and older), OCD (7 and older), PMDD, bulimia, panic disorder.

Common Side Effects: GI upset, sexual dysfunction, insomnia, agitation, headache, and nausea, which should improve in 3 to 5 days.

Rare: *Seizures, hyponatremia, induction of mania, and activation of suicidal ideation in those under 24.*

Monitoring: ECG if QT prolongation. Height and weight on children.

Pearl: There is no need to taper due to long half-life.

Contraindications: Taking MAO-I, thioridazine, pimozide, or tamoxifen.

Black Box Warning: Use may increase suicidal thoughts in children, adolescents, and young adults (24 and younger) [19].

Paroxetine (Paxil)

Starting Dose: Immediate Release: 20 mg PO daily. 10 mg PO daily can be used in the elderly.

Controlled Release: 25 mg PO daily.

Titration: Immediate Release: Increase by 10 mg PO daily every week.

Controlled Release: 12.5 mg po daily. Wait for 4–6 weeks for the response when initializing therapy.

Max Dose: Immediate Release: 50 mg PO daily.

Controlled Release: 62.5 mg PO daily.

FDA Approval: MDD, OCD, panic disorder, SAD, PTSD, GAD, PMDD.

Common Side Effects: GI upset, sexual dysfunction, agitation, headache, and nausea, which should improve in 3–5 days.

Rare: *Seizures, hyponatremia, induction of mania, and activation of suicidal ideation in those under 24.*

Pearl: There is a need to wean over several months for those who cannot tolerate withdrawal effects.

Contraindications: Taking MAO-I, thioridazine, pimozide, or tamoxifen.

Black Box Warning: Use may increase suicidal thoughts in children, adolescents, and young adults (24 and younger) [10, 11].

*****Beers List for drugs to avoid in the elderly*****

Sertraline (Zoloft)

Starting Dose: 50 mg PO daily. 25 mg PO daily in elderly.

Titration: Increase by 25–50 mg PO daily every week. Wait for 4–6 weeks for the response when initializing therapy.

Max Dose: 200 mg PO daily.

FDA Approval: Major depressive disorder (MDD), obsessive compulsive disorder (OCD), panic disorder, posttraumatic stress disorder (PTSD), premenstrual dysphoric disorder (PMDD), social anxiety disorder (SAD).

Common Side Effects: GI upset, sexual dysfunction, agitation, headache, and nausea, which should improve in 3–5 days.

Rare: *Seizures, hyponatremia, induction of mania, hypotension, and activation of suicidal ideation in those under 24.*

Contraindications: Taking MAO-I, thioridazine, pimozide, or tamoxifen. Do not use Zoloft oral concentrate if the patient is taking disulfiram.

Black Box Warning: Use may increase suicidal thoughts in children, adolescents, and young adults (24 and younger) [15, 16].

Venlafaxine XR (Effexor XR)

Starting Dose: 37.5 mg PO daily.

Titration: Increase by 37.5 mg PO daily in 1 week. Then, titrate by 75 mg PO daily. Wait for 4–6 weeks (on 75 mg dose) for the response when initializing therapy.

Max Dose: 375 mg PO daily.

FDA Approval: Depression, GAD, SAD, panic disorder, separation anxiety disorder.

Common Side Effects: INCREASED blood pressure, GI upset, sexual dysfunction, insomnia, agitation, anxiety, sweating, headache, and nausea, which should improve in 3–5 days.

Rare: *Seizures, hyponatremia, induction of mania, and activation of suicidal ideation in those under 24.*

Monitoring: Blood pressure at each visit.

Pearls: Higher doses are associated with more side effects. Immediate release forms are available but are more prone to discontinuation syndrome. Effexor can be difficult to wean; alternative strategies may need to be used and length of titration may take months. Patients commonly report “brain zaps” while discontinuing or even missing a dose.

Contraindications: Taking MAO-I, thioridazine, pimozide, or tamoxifen.

Black Box Warning: Use may increase suicidal thoughts in children, adolescents, and young adults (24 and younger) [12].

*** All other SSRIs and antidepressants are considered off label but are equally efficacious. ***

A Note About Benzodiazepines

Benzodiazepines are considered second-line treatments. There is an increased risk of substance abuse associated with benzodiazepines. They should be used in lowest effective dose for the shortest amount of time possible. Typically, it is used as a bridge therapy while waiting for efficacy of first-line treatments. Familiarize yourself with one drug in each category and become comfortable prescribing it. Remember that short-acting benzos will more likely cause withdrawal effects and long-acting benzos can build up in a patient's system, especially the elderly.

*****Beers List for drugs to avoid in the elderly*****

Adjunctive Medications: Panic Disorder

Alprazolam (Xanax)

Starting Dose: 0.25 mg PO (Daily to TID) PRN.

Titration: 0.25 mg to 0.5 mg PO (Daily to TID).

Max Dose: 3 mg/day.

FDA Approval: Generalized anxiety disorder and panic disorder.

Off-Label Disorders: Other anxiety disorders, anxiety associated with depression, IBS, acute mania, acute psychosis, and catatonia.

Common Side Effects: Sedation, fatigue, depression, dizziness, ataxia, slurred speech, weakness, forgetfulness, confusion, hyperexcitability, nervousness, dry mouth, mania, hypotension, *respiratory depression.*

Rare: Hepatic dysfunction, renal dysfunction, blood dyscrasias.

Pearl: Withdrawal may occur with prolonged use, and patients will need expert guidance on discontinuing medication. DO NOT MIX WITH ALCOHOL.

Contraindicated: Angle-closure glaucoma or with concomitant azole use [15, 16].

Clonazepam (Klonopin)

Starting Dose: 0.25 mg PO (Daily to BID) PRN.

Titration: 0.25 mg to 0.5 mg PO (Daily) PRN.

Max Dose: 4 mg/day.

FDA Approval: Panic disorder, Lennox-Gastaut syndrome, akinetic seizure, myoclonic seizure, and absence seizure.

Off-Label Disorders: Atonic seizures, other anxiety disorders, insomnia, and catatonia.

Common Side Effects: Sedation, fatigue, depression, dizziness, ataxia, slurred speech, weakness, forgetfulness, confusion, hyperexcitability, nervousness, dry mouth, mania, hypotension, *respiratory depression.*

Rare: *Hepatic dysfunction, renal dysfunction, blood dyscrasias.*

Pearl: Withdrawal can occur with prolonged use, and the patient will need expert guidance on discontinuing medication. DO NOT MIX WITH ALCOHOL.

Contraindicated: Angle-closure glaucoma or with concomitant azole use [20].

Social Anxiety Disorder

Social anxiety disorder (SAD), also known as social phobia, is a condition hallmarked by intense fear or anxiety related to certain social situations. The fear and anxiety is related to the feeling that one will be judged, embarrassed, or humiliated in certain social contexts. It can occur during job interviews, in a classroom setting, having to speak in public, or eating in public, among many other instances. The fear and anxiety the person feels is always disproportionate to the actual situation.

FEARED: **F**ear of social situations where exposed to possible scrutiny by others/**F**ears of being negatively evaluated, **E**xposure to the social situation almost always provokes fear or anxiety, **A**voids the social situation or endured with intense fear or anxiety, **R**ecognizes that the fear is out of proportion, **E**xclusion of fear induced by a substance or another mental or medical disorder, **D**uration lasting for 6 months [1].

DSM-5-TR

The DSM-5-TR lists social anxiety disorder as a disorder that causes heightened anxiety or fear about social situations where other people may negatively evaluate the patient. Examples are school settings, being in an area where they may be observed, or giving a presentation. The patient fears they will be "negatively evaluated" or embarrass themselves. The situations almost always provoke the anxiety or fear. Patients will typically avoid the situations if possible or be under extreme duress if they must be there. The fear is persistent for at least 6 months and is out of proportion to the threat posed. The anxiety is not the result of a physiological effect, drug, or other medical condition. It cannot be better explained by another mental illness [2, p. 229].

Differential Diagnosis: Autism, depression, generalized anxiety, intermittent explosive disorder, panic disorder.

Screening Scales

Social Phobia Inventory (SPIN): It is a self-reported scale that consists of 17 items covering the spectrum of social phobia. Each item is ranked on a scale of intensity, from "Not at All" to "Extremely," and assigned a corresponding number value. A score higher than 19 indicates likelihood of a social anxiety disorder.

Social Phobia and Anxiety Inventory (SPAI): It is a 45-item test that assesses specific somatic symptoms, cognitions, and behaviors across a wide range of fear-producing situations to measure social anxiety and fear.

Treatment

Treatment of SAD should be based on patient preference and availability of therapy options. Cognitive behavioral therapy and pharmacotherapy have shown similar efficacy, but there is a lack of evidence showing combining modalities is the superior approach. There is limited evidence showing superiority of one SSRI over the other, but all of the FDA-approved medications will be listed below [21].

Non-pharmacological Treatments: Cognitive behavioral therapy, exposure therapy, and relaxation therapy [21]..

First-Line Medications: Social Anxiety Disorder

Fluvoxamine CR (Luvox CR)

Starting Dose: 100 mg PO nightly.

Titration: Increase by 100 mg PO nightly every week.

Max Dose: 300 mg PO daily.

FDA Approval: Obsessive compulsive disorder and social anxiety disorder.

Common Side Effects: GI upset, sexual dysfunction, sweating, insomnia, agitation, headache, and nausea, which should improve in 3–5 days.

Rare: *Seizures, hyponatremia, induction of mania, and activation of suicidal ideation in those under 24.*

Monitoring: None.

Pearl: Usually given at night due to sedation. Doses greater than 100 mg can be twice daily dosing to improve tolerability.

Contraindications: Taking MAO-I, thioridazine, pimozide, or tamoxifen.

Black Box Warning: Use may increase suicidal thoughts in children, adolescents, and young adults (24 and younger) [22].

Paroxetine (Paxil)

Starting Dose:

Immediate Release: 20 mg PO daily. 10 mg PO daily can be used in elderly.

Controlled Release: 25 mg PO daily.

Titration:

Immediate Release: Increase by 10 mg PO daily, after 1 week. Wait for 4–6 weeks for the response when initializing therapy.

Controlled Release: 12.5 mg po daily, after 1 week. Wait for 4–6 weeks for the response when initializing therapy.

Max Dose:

Immediate Release: 50 mg PO daily.

Controlled Release: 62.5 mg po daily.

FDA Approval: MDD, OCD, panic disorder, SAD, PTSD, GAD, PMDD.

Common Side Effects: GI upset, sexual dysfunction, agitation, headache, sedation, dizziness, tremor, bruising, weight gain, and nausea, which should improve in 3–5 days.

Rare: *Seizures, hyponatremia, induction of mania, Serotonin Syndrome, bleeding, SIADH, and activation of suicidal ideation in those under 24.*

Pearl: There is a need to wean over several months for those who cannot tolerate withdrawal effects.

Contraindications: Taking MAO-I, thioridazine, pimozide, or tamoxifen.

Black Box Warning: Use may increase suicidal thoughts in children, adolescents, and young adults (24 and younger) [10, 11].

*****Beers List for drugs to avoid in the elderly*****

Sertraline (Zoloft)

Starting Dose: 50 mg PO daily. 25 mg PO daily in elderly.

Titration: Increase by 25–50 mg PO daily every week. Wait for 4–6 weeks for the response when initializing therapy.

Max Dose: 200 mg PO daily.

FDA Approval: Major depressive disorder (MDD), obsessive compulsive disorder (OCD), panic disorder, posttraumatic stress disorder (PTSD), premenstrual dysphoric disorder (PMDD), social anxiety disorder.

Common Side Effects: GI upset, sexual dysfunction, agitation, headache, insomnia, sedation, sweating, bruising, and nausea, which should improve in 3–5 days.

Rare: *Seizures, hyponatremia, induction of mania, hypotension, Serotonin Syndrome, bleeding, SIADH, and activation of suicidal ideation in those under 24.*

Contraindications: Taking MAO-I, thioridazine, pimozide, or tamoxifen.

Black Box Warning: Use may increase suicidal thoughts in children, adolescents, and young adults (24 and younger) [15, 16].

Venlafaxine XR (Effexor XR)

Starting Dose: 37.5 mg PO daily.

Titration: Increase by 37.5 mg PO daily in 1 week. Then, titrate by 75 mg PO daily. Wait for 4–6 weeks (on 75 mg dose) for the response when initializing therapy.

Max Dose: 375 mg PO daily.

FDA Approval: Depression, GAD, SAD, panic disorder, separation anxiety disorder.

Common Side Effects: INCREASED blood pressure, GI upset, sexual dysfunction, insomnia, agitation, anxiety, sweating, abnormal vision, headache, and nausea, which should improve in 3–5 days.

Rare: *Seizures, hyponatremia, induction of mania, Serotonin Syndrome, SIADH, and activation of suicidal ideation in those under 24.*

Monitoring: Blood pressure at each visit.

Pearls: Higher doses are associated with more side effects. Immediate release forms are available but are more prone to discontinuation syndrome. Effexor can be difficult to wean; alternative strategies may need to be used and length of titration may take months. Patients commonly report "brain zaps" while discontinuing or even missing a dose. Medication is renally cleared and may need dose reduction of 25–50% in renal disease.

Contraindications: Uncontrolled angle-closure glaucoma or taking a MAO-I.

Black Box Warning: Use may increase suicidal thoughts in children, adolescents, and young adults (24 and younger) [12].

*** All other SSRIs and antidepressants are considered off label but are equally efficacious. ***

Treatment-Resistant Anxiety

A significant portion of patients with GAD will not find relief from available FDA-approved medications. Sometimes it is necessary to explore secondary options. While this is best left to seasoned prescribers, the following medications have found some efficacy in treatment-resistant anxiety disorders. If you find yourself going down this pathway, it would be prudent to refer to a seasoned psychiatric provider.

Off-Label Use for Treatment-Resistant Anxiety

Gabapentin (Neurontin)

Starting Dose: 100 mg PO BID.

Titration: Increase by 300–600 mg daily every 4–7 days.

Max Dose: Not much more benefit above 600 mg PO TID.

FDA Approval: Partial seizures, postherpetic neuralgia, restless leg syndrome (extended release).

Off-Label Anxiety Disorders: Anxiety.

Common Side Effects: Sedation, dizziness, ataxia, peripheral edema, blurred vision, GI upset, heartburn, and dry mouth.

Rare: *Activation of suicidal ideation, anaphylaxis*, and *angioedema*.

Monitoring: GAD-7, monitor for sedation.

Pearl: Do not take antacid within 2 h of taking gabapentin. Taper over a minimum of 1 week [23, 24].

Olanzapine (Zyprexa)

Starting Dose: 2.5–5 mg PO nightly.

Titration: 2.5 mg PO nightly every week.

Max Dose: 5 mg to 7.5 mg for anxiety.

FDA Approval: Treatment-resistant depression, schizophrenia, bipolar maintenance, bipolar depression.

Common Side Effects: Increased risk for diabetes and dyslipidemia, dizziness, sedation, dry mouth, constipation, weight gain, edema, musculoskeletal pain, orthostatic hypotension, tardive dyskinesia.

Rare: *DRESS*, *hyperglycemia (ketoacidosis)*, *NMS*, *seizures.*

Monitoring: GAD-7, BMI every 3 months, lipid panel, and A1c annually. Waist circumference, blood pressure, fasting plasma glucose, and fasting lipid profile prior to start, within 3 months, and then annually. AIMS score every 6 months to 1 year.

Pearl: Patient maybe given prn in ½ tablets of 2.5 mg tablets.

Contraindications: Risk of angle-closure glaucoma, unstable cardiac condition.

Black Box Warning: Elderly dementia patients who take Zyprexa have a higher risk of death. Use may increase suicidal thoughts in children, adolescents, and young adults (24 and younger) [25].

> *****Beers List for drugs to avoid in the elderly*****

Pregabalin (Lyrica)

Starting Dose: 75 mg PO BID, 150 mg/day.

Titration: Increase by 150 mg/day weekly—BID or TID dosing.

Max Dose: 600 mg PO daily.

FDA Approval: Diabetic peripheral neuropathy, postherpetic neuralgia, neuropathic pain r/t spinal cord injury, and partial onset seizures.

Off-Label Anxiety Disorders: GAD, panic disorder, social anxiety disorder.

Common Side Effects: Sedation, dizziness, dry mouth, impaired attention, ataxia, fatigue, blurred vision, peripheral edema, diplopia, decreased libido, erectile dysfunction, tremor, irritability, GI upset, and weight gain.

Rare: *Activation of suicidal ideation.*

Monitoring: GAD-7.

Pearl: If given with additional sedating medication, titrate slowly after 1 week. It is better tolerated with TID dosing.

Contraindication: Galactose intolerance, the Lapp lactase deficiency, or glucose-galactose malabsorption [23, 24].

Quetiapine XR (Seroquel XR)

Starting Dose: 50 mg PO nightly.

Titration: Increase by 50 mg to 100 mg PO nightly.

Max Dose: Usually 150 mg for anxiety.

FDA Approval: MDD, bipolar depression, bipolar maintenance, schizophrenia.

Common Side Effects: GI upset, sexual dysfunction, insomnia, agitation, sedation, dizziness, urinary retention, headache, weight loss, myalgia, sweating, anorexia, hypertension, and nausea better in 3–5 days.

Rare: *Neuroleptic malignant syndrome, seizures.*

Monitoring: PHQ-9, BMI every 3 months, lipid panel, and A1c annually. Waist circumference, blood pressure, fasting plasma glucose, and fasting lipid profile prior to start, within 3 months, and then annually. AIMS score every 3 to 6 months.

Pearl: Known for sedating properties, it could be a useful insomnia adjunct in doses up to 100 mg.

Black Box Warning: Elderly dementia patients who take Seroquel have a higher risk of death. Use may increase suicidal thoughts in children, adolescents, and young adults (24 and younger) [26].

*****Beers List for drugs to avoid in the elderly*****

A Note About Benzodiazepines

Benzodiazepines are considered second-line treatments. There is an increased risk of substance abuse associated with benzodiazepines. They should be used in the lowest effective dose for the shortest amount of time possible. Typically, it is used as a bridge therapy while waiting for efficacy of first-line treatments. Familiarize yourself with one drug in each category and become comfortable prescribing it. Remember that short-acting benzos will more likely cause withdrawal effects and long-acting benzos can build up in a patient's system, especially the elderly.

*****Beers List for drugs to avoid in the elderly*****

Short-acting benzos	Alprazolam and oxazepam
Intermediate-acting benzos	Lorazepam and clonazepam
Long-acting benzos	Clorazepate, diazepam, and flurazepam
Benzos safe in liver disease	Oxazepam, temazepam (insomnia), and lorazepam

Alprazolam (Xanax)

Starting Dose: 0.25 mg PO TID PRN.

Titration: 0.25 mg to 0.5 mg PO TID.

Max Dose: 3 mg.

FDA Approval: Diabetic generalized anxiety disorder, panic disorder.

Off-Label Disorders: Other anxiety disorders, anxiety associated with depression, IBS, acute mania, acute psychosis, and catatonia.

Common Side Effects: Sedation, fatigue, depression, dizziness, ataxia, slurred speech, weakness, forgetfulness, confusion, hyperexcitability, nervousness, dry mouth, mania, hypotension, *respiratory depression.*

Rare: *Hepatic dysfunction, renal dysfunction, blood dyscrasias.*

Monitoring: GAD-7.

Pearl: Withdrawal can occur with prolonged use, and patient will need expert guidance on discontinuing medication.

Contraindicated: Angle-closure glaucoma or with concomitant azole use [15, 16].

Clonazepam (Klonopin)

Starting Dose: 0.25 mg PO (Daily to BID) PRN.

Titration: 0.25 mg to 0.5 mg PO (Daily) PRN.

Max Dose: 4 mg/day.

FDA Approval: Panic disorder, Lennox-Gastaut syndrome, akinetic seizure, myoclonic seizure, and absence of seizure.

Off-Label Disorders: Atonic seizures, other anxiety disorders, insomnia, and catatonia.

Common Side Effects: Sedation, fatigue, depression, dizziness, ataxia, slurred speech, weakness, forgetfulness, confusion, hyperexcitability, nervousness, dry mouth, mania, hypotension, *respiratory depression.*

Rare: *Hepatic dysfunction, renal dysfunction, blood dyscrasias.*

Monitoring: GAD-7.

Pearl: Withdrawal can occur with prolonged use, and patient will need expert guidance on discontinuing medication. DO NOT MIX WITH ALCOHOL.

Contraindicated: Angle-closure glaucoma or with concomitant azole use [20].

Clorazepate (Tranxene)

Starting Dose: 7.5 mg PO BID—15 mg/day.

Titration: 7.5 mg PO TID.

Max Dose: 90 mg/day.

FDA Approval: Anxiety disorder, symptoms of anxiety, acute alcohol withdrawal.

Off-Label Disorders: Partial seizures and catatonia.

Common Side Effects: Sedation, fatigue, depression, dizziness, ataxia, slurred speech, weakness, forgetfulness, confusion, hyperexcitability, nervousness, dry mouth, mania, hypotension, and *respiratory depression*.

Rare: *Hepatic dysfunction, renal dysfunction, blood dyscrasias.*

Monitoring: GAD-7.

Pearl: Withdrawal can occur with prolonged use, and patient will need expert guidance on discontinuing medication.

Contraindicated in angle-closure glaucoma [27].

Lorazepam (Ativan)

Starting Dose: 2 mg/day broken down into TID dosing.

Titration: 0.5 mg PO TID or 1.5 mg daily.

Max Dose: 10 mg/day.

FDA Approval: Anxiety disorder, anxiety associated with depressive symptoms, status epilepticus, preanesthetic.

Off-Label Disorders: Insomnia, alcohol withdrawal psychosis, panic disorder, acute mania, acute psychosis, catatonia.

Common Side Effects: Sedation, fatigue, depression, dizziness, ataxia, slurred speech, weakness, forgetfulness, confusion, hyperexcitability, nervousness, dry mouth, mania, hypotension, *respiratory depression.*

Rare: *Hepatic dysfunction, renal dysfunction, blood dyscrasias.*

Monitoring: GAD-7.

Pearl: Withdrawal can occur with prolonged use, and patient will need expert guidance on discontinuing medication.

Contraindicated: Angle-closure glaucoma or with concomitant azole use [28].

Oxazepam (Serax)

Starting Dose: Mild to Moderate: 10–15 mg PO TID/QID. Range: 30–60 mg/day.
Severe: Up to 30 mg PO TID/QID. Range: 45–120 mg/day

Titration: Titration is usually not necessary.

Max Dose: 120 mg/day.

FDA Approval: Anxiety, anxiety associated with depression, and alcohol withdrawal.

Off-Label Disorders: Catatonia.

Common Side Effects: Sedation, fatigue, depression, dizziness, ataxia, slurred speech, weakness, forgetfulness, confusion, hyperexcitability, nervousness, dry mouth, mania, hypotension, *respiratory depression.*

Rare: *Hepatic dysfunction, renal dysfunction, blood dyscrasias.*

Monitoring: GAD-7.

Pearl: Withdrawal can occur with prolonged use, and patient will need expert guidance on discontinuing medication.

Contraindicated: Angle-closure glaucoma or with concomitant azole use [29].

References

1. Caplan J, Stern T. Mnemonics in a mnutshell: 32 aids to psychiatric diagnosis. Curr Psychiatr Ther. 2008;7(10):27–33.
2. American Psychiatric Association. Anxiety disorders. In: Diagnostic and statistical manual of mental disorders (5th-TR). Washington, DC: American Psychiatric Association; 2022.
3. Bhatt NV. Anxiety disorders differential diagnoses; 2024, March 19. Retrieved April 5, 2024, from https://emedicine.medscape.com/article/286227-differential?form=fpf.
4. Meek W, PhD. Generalized anxiety disorder: causes and risk factors. Very well Mind; 2021, October 12. https://www.verywellmind.com/gad-causes-risk-factors-1392982.
5. Spitzer RL, Kroenke K, Williams JBW, Lowe B. A brief measure for assessing generalized anxiety disorder. Arch Inern Med. 2006;166:1092–7.
6. Hamilton M. The assessment of anxiety states by rating. Br J Med Psychol. 1959;32:50–5.

7. Craske M, Bystritsky A. UpToDate; 2024, March 28. UpToDate. Retrieved April 5, 2024, from https://www.uptodate.com/contents/generalized-anxiety-disorder-in-adults-management.
8. Eli Lilly and Company. Cymbalta: highlights of prescribing information; 2023. https://pi.lilly.com/us/cymbalta-pi.pdf.
9. Forest Pharmaceuticals, Inc. Lexapro: highlights of prescribing information; 2009. https://www.accessdata.fda.gov/drugsatfda_docs/label/2009/021323s030s031,021365s021s022lbl.pdf.
10. GlaxoSmithKline. Paxil: prescribing information; 2008. https://www.accessdata.fda.gov/drugsatfda_docs/label/2008/020031s060,020936s037,020710s024lbl.pdf.
11. GlaxoSmithKline. Paxil CR: prescribing information; 2014. https://www.accessdata.fda.gov/drugsatfda_docs/label/2014/020936s049lbl.pdf.
12. Viatris Specialty LLC. Effexor XR: highlights of prescribing information; 2023. https://www.accessdata.fda.gov/drugsatfda_docs/label/2023/020699s118lbl.pdf.
13. Bristol-Myers Squibb Company. Buspar: prescribing information; 2000. https://www.accessdata.fda.gov/drugsatfda_docs/label/2001/18731s43lbl.pdf.
14. Pfizer Inc. Vistaril: medical information; 2023. https://www.pfizermedicalinformation.com/en-us/vistaril.
15. Pfizer Inc. Xanax: highlights of prescribing information; 2021. https://www.accessdata.fda.gov/drugsatfda_docs/label/2021/018276s055lbl.pdf.
16. Pfizer Inc. Zoloft: highlights of prescribing information; 2021. https://labeling.pfizer.com/ShowLabeling.aspx?id=517.
17. Forrest JS. Pediatric panic disorder differential diagnoses; 2018, October 4. https://emedicine.medscape.com/article/914490-differential.
18. Panic Disorder Screener (PADIS) | National Centre for Epidemiology and Population Health; n.d. https://nceph.anu.edu.au/research/tools-resources/panic-disorder-screener-padis.
19. Eli Lilly and Company. Prozac: highlights of prescribing information; 1987. https://pi.lilly.com/us/prozac.pdf.
20. Genentech, Inc. Klonopin: prescribing information; 2013. https://www.accessdata.fda.gov/drugsatfda_docs/label/2013/017533s053,020813s009lbl.pdf.
21. Social anxiety disorder: more than just shyness. (n.d). National Institute of Mental Health (NIMH). https://www.nimh.nih.gov/health/publications/social-anxiety-disorder-more-than-just-shyness.
22. Jazz Pharmaceuticals. Luvox CR: highlights of prescribing information; 2008. https://www.accessdata.fda.gov/drugsatfda_docs/label/2009/022033s002lbl.pdf.
23. Pfizer Inc. Lyrica: highlights of prescribing information; 2020. https://labeling.pfizer.com/showlabeling.aspx?id=561.

24. Pfizer Inc. Neurontin: highlights of prescribing information; 2020. https://www.accessdata.fda.gov/drugsatfda_docs/label/2021/018276s055lbl.pdf.
25. Eli Lilly and Company. Zyprexa: highlights of prescribing information; 2021. https://pi.lilly.com/us/zyprexa-pi.pdf.
26. AstraZeneca Pharmaceuticals LP. Seroquel XR: highlights of prescribing information; 2009. https://www.accessdata.fda.gov/drugsatfda_docs/label/2009/022047s011s016s017s019s022lbl.pdf.
27. Abbott Pharmaceuticals PR Ltd. Tranxene: prescribing information; 2010. https://www.accessdata.fda.gov/drugsatfda_docs/label/2010/017105s076lbl.pdf.
28. Bausch Health Companies Inc. Ativan: prescribing information; 2022. https://www.accessdata.fda.gov/drugsatfda_docs/label/2023/017794s049lbl.pdf.
29. Singh R, Abdijadid S. Oxazepam. StatPearls - NCBI Bookshelf; 2023, May 22. https://www.ncbi.nlm.nih.gov/books/NBK544349/

Attention Deficit Hyperactivity Disorder (ADHD)

3

Contents

Adult Attention Deficit Hyperactivity Disorder

Attention deficit hyperactivity disorder (ADHD) is a neurodevelopmental disorder that typically first manifests between the ages of 6 and 12 years old. It is hallmarked by inattentiveness, difficulty concentrating, impulsive behavior, and in many cases hyperactivity. The hyperactivity component tends to improve into adulthood, but inattentiveness may remain. While ADHD is a childhood disorder, many adults have lived with it their entire life without a diagnosis until later in their life.

B. Floyd, T. Kane, *The Clinician's Guide to Common Psychiatric Disorders*, https://doi.org/10.1007/978-3-031-67958-2_3

Diagnosing and Monitoring

Mnemonic

DISTRACTED: **D**istractibility, **I**mpulsivity, **S**chool history, **T**ask completion, **R**ating scales, **A**ccidents, **C**ommitments, **T**ime management, **E**mployment, **D**ecisions, hasty [1].

Diagnosis

Most adult patients will come to the provider with an ADHD diagnosis and will be continuing care. For adults without an ADHD diagnosis that want to be evaluated, it is good practice to offer them neuropsychological testing from a trained, certified psychologist. ADHD is an adolescent onset disorder so symptoms should be present since childhood. See the DSM-5-TR for full criteria.

Differential Diagnosis: Under stimulated home environment, substance abuse, major depressive disorder, personality disorders, bipolar, generalized anxiety disorder, mild autism, obsessive compulsive disorder, oppositional defiance disorder, conduct disorder, and stereotypic movement disorder [2].

Risk Factors: Genetic loading, pregnancy and perinatal complications, family conflict, low birth weight, neglect/foster placement, alcohol exposure in utero, reduced behavioral inhibition [3].

Labs to Consider: Nonspecific.

Screening Scales

Adult ADHD Self-Report Scale (ASRS) v1.1: It is a two-part symptom checklist with Part A consisting of 6 questions and Part B consisting of 12 questions. Patient rates each symptom by how often they are bothered by it from "never" to "very often." If four questions on Part A are in the shaded boxes, it is highly consistent with ADHD. The shaded boxes of Part B will help the clinician further explore bothersome symptoms.

ADHD Rating Scale IV (ADHD-RS-IV) with Adult Prompts: There are 18 question survey asking about adult ADHD symptom's frequency and severity. Nine questions cover inattentiveness, while the other nine cover hyperactivity. Answers are rated on a frequency scale from 0 (Never) to 3 (Very Often).

Treatment

Treatment should consist of pharmacological and non-pharmacological treatment in order to have the most robust response. Psychotherapies that have shown benefit for ADHD are lacking. However, cognitive behavioral therapy (CBT) that targets executive dysfunction has been shown to be helpful for patients who still struggle with time management and organization. Other non-pharmacological interventions include cognitive behavioral training programs, psychoeducation, and treating comorbid learning disorders [4].

First-line pharmacological treatment for ADHD is stimulant medications over nonstimulant as nonstimulant medications typically take up to 4 weeks to provide any benefit and stimulants can provide a benefit almost immediately. Preferred stimulants are those within the amphetamine group vs methylphenidate, although both provide benefit. It should be noted that amphetamines may have higher abuse potential.

Non-pharmacologic Interventions

Cognitive Behavioral Therapy Targeting Executive Function: It is a therapy that helps identify negative thought patterns and teaches the patient how to restructure negative thoughts so they become positive thought processes. CBT for ADHD also includes strategies to help with distractibility delay, guided discovery, and successive approximation.

Pharmacologic Interventions

Nonstimulant ADHD Medications

Atomoxetine (Strattera)
Starting Dose: 40 mg PO daily.

Titration: Increase to 80 mg after 7 days and then to 100 mg PO daily in 2–4 weeks.

Max Dose: 100 mg/day.

FDA Approval: ADHD in children 6 and older.

Common Side Effects: Sedation, fatigue, decreased appetite, increased heart rate and blood pressure, insomnia, dizziness, irritability, dry mouth, constipation, nausea, vomiting, abdominal pain, heartburn, sexual dysfunction, anxiety, agitation, and aggression.

Rare: *Cardiovascular adverse effects, severe liver damage, hypomania, priapism, activation of suicidal ideation.*

Monitoring: Blood pressure at initiation, after dose increase, and periodically.

Contraindications: Taking a MAO-I, history of pheochromocytoma, severe cardiovascular disorder, angle-closure glaucoma.

Black Box Warning: Use may increase the risk of suicidality in children/adolescents with ADHD, especially within the first month of treatment [5].

Clonidine (Kapvay): Ages 6–17

Starting Dose: Extended Release: 0.1 mg PO nightly.

Titration: Extended Release: 0.1 mg per week, after 3–4 weeks.

Max Dose: Extended Release: 4 mg.

FDA Approval: Hypertension, ADHD in children 6–17 years old.

Common Side Effects: Sedation, dizziness, abdominal pain, nausea, fatigue, weakness, hypotension, dry mouth, constipation, and bradycardia.

Rare: *Sinus bradycardia, atrioventricular block, hypertensive encephalopathy, CVA, and death* (during withdrawal).

Monitoring: Blood pressure regularly [6].

*****Beers List for drugs to avoid in the elderly*****

Guanfacine (Intuniv): Ages 6–17

Starting Dose: Extended Release: 1 mg PO daily.

Titration: Extended Release: Increase by 1 mg PO daily every week.

Max Dose: 4 mg/day.

FDA Approval: Hypertension, ADHD in children 6–17 years old.

Common Side Effects: Dry mouth, constipation, hypotension, insomnia, agitation, dizziness, lightheadedness, headache, fatigue, blurred vision, nausea, orthostatic hypotension, *sinus bradycardia*.

Monitoring: None.

Pearl: Given during the day for hyperarousal, not typically given to treat nightmares [7].

*****Beers List for drugs to avoid in the elderly*****

Viloxazine (Qelbree) (12 years old +)

Starting Dose: 200 mg PO daily.

Titration: Increase 200 mg PO daily each week.

Max Dose: 600 mg/day, Ages 12–17: 400 mg/day.

FDA Approval: ADHD ages 6 and up.

Common Side Effects: Fatigue, sleepiness, insomnia, irritability, headache, decreased appetite, nausea, vomiting, dry mouth, constipation, increased heart rate and blood pressure.

Rare: *Hypomania*.

Monitoring: Blood pressure at initiation, after dose increase, and periodically throughout treatment.

Contraindications: Taking MAOI inhibitor, history of pheochromocytoma, angle-closure glaucoma, and severe cardiovascular disorder.

Pearl: If too sedating, take at night to reduce daytime drowsiness.

Black Box Warning: Use may increase the risk of suicidality in children/adolescents with ADHD, especially within first month of treatment [8].

Stimulant Medications

There are numerous stimulant preparations each with varying half-life and dosage instructions. Below are some of the most common. Recommendation is to pick several that you are comfortable with and get used to prescribing them.

Amphetamine, d, (Dexedrine)

Starting Dose: 5 mg PO BID.

Titration: Increase by 5–10 mg PO BID each week.

Max Dose: 60 mg/day,

FDA Approval: ADHD ages 6 and up.

Common Side Effects: Insomnia, headache, exacerbation of tics, nervousness, irritability, overstimulation, tremor, dizziness, anorexia, dry mouth, nausea, diarrhea, constipation, sexual dysfunction if used long term.

Uncommon: *Psychotic episodes, seizures, palpitations, cardiovascular adverse effects.*

Monitoring: Assess for cardiac disease before initiation. Blood pressure and heart rate should be monitored regularly. Monitor height and weight in children.

Contraindications: Extreme anxiety, motor tics, taking a MAOI, patient has history of arteriosclerosis, cardiovascular disease, severe hypertension, glaucoma, structural cardiac abnormalities, cardiomyopathy, serious heart arrythmias, or CAD.

Black Box Warning: High abuse potential [9].

Amphetamine, d, l (Adderall, Adderall XR)

Starting Dose: 5 mg PO BID, Extended Release: 12.5 mg PO upon waking.

Titration: Increase by 5–10 mg PO BID each week. Extended Release: Increase by 12.5 mg PO daily every week.

Max Dose: 40 mg/day, Extended Release: 50 mg/day.

FDA Approval: ADHD ages 6 and up. Narcolepsy in patients 6 and up. Exogenous obesity in ages 12 and up.

Common Side Effects: Insomnia, headache, exacerbation of tics, nervousness, irritability, overstimulation, tremor, dizziness, anorexia, dry mouth, nausea, diarrhea, constipation, long-term sexual dysfunction.

Uncommon: *Psychotic episodes, seizures, palpitations, cardiovascular adverse effects.*

Monitoring: Assess for cardiac disease before initiation. Blood pressure and heart rate should be monitored regularly. Monitor height and weight in children.

Contraindications: Extreme anxiety, motor tics, taking a MAOI, patient has history of arteriosclerosis, cardiovascular disease, severe hypertension, glaucoma, structural cardiac abnormalities, cardiomyopathy, serious heart arrythmias, or CAD.

Black Box Warning: High abuse potential [10, 11].

Lisdexamfetamine (Vyvanse)

Starting Dose: 30 mg PO daily.

Titration: Increase 10–20 mg PO daily every week.

Max Dose: 70 mg/day.

FDA Approval: ADHD ages 6 and up. Binge eating disorder.

Common Side Effects: Fatigue, sleepiness, insomnia, irritability, headache, decreased appetite, nausea, vomiting, dry mouth, constipation, increased heart rate and blood pressure,

Uncommon: *Psychotic episodes, seizures, palpitations, tachycardia, hypertension, cardiovascular adverse effects.*

Rare: *Activation of hypomania.*

Monitoring: Blood pressure at initiation, after dose increase, and periodically throughout treatment.

Contraindications: Taking MAOI inhibitor, history of pheochromocytoma, angle-closure glaucoma, hyperthyroidism, and severe cardiovascular disorder.

Pearl: Taper to avoid withdrawal effects.

Black Box Warning: High abuse potential [12].

Methylphenidate d (Focalin)

Starting Dose: 2.5 mg PO BID,

Titration: Increase by 2.5–5 mg/day every week.

Max Dose: 10 mg BID.

FDA Approval: ADHD ages 6–17.

Common Side Effects: Insomnia, headache, exacerbation of tics, nervousness, irritability, overstimulation, tremor, dizziness, anorexia, dry mouth, nausea.

Uncommon: *Psychotic episodes, seizures, palpitations, priapism, and cardiovascular adverse effects.*

Monitoring: Assess for cardiac disease before initiation. Blood pressure and heart rate should be monitored regularly. Monitor height and weight in children.

Contraindications: Extreme anxiety, motor tics, taking a MAOI, cardiovascular disease, glaucoma, structural cardiac abnormalities, cardiomyopathy, serious heart arrythmias, or CAD.

Black Box Warning: High abuse potential [13].

Methylphenidate d Extended Release Capsules (Focalin XR)

Starting Dose: 10 mg PO daily,

Titration: Increase by 10 mg/day, after 1 week.

Max Dose: 40 mg daily.

FDA Approval: ADHD ages 6–17. ADHD in adults.

Common Side Effects: Insomnia, headache, exacerbation of tics, nervousness, irritability, overstimulation, tremor, dizziness, anorexia, dry mouth, nausea.

Uncommon: *Psychotic episodes, seizures, palpitations, priapism, and cardiovascular adverse effects.*

Monitoring: Assess for cardiac disease before initiation. Blood pressure and heart rate should be monitored regularly. Monitor height and weight in children.

Contraindications: Extreme anxiety, motor tics, taking a MAOI, cardiovascular disease, glaucoma, structural cardiac abnormalities, cardiomyopathy, serious heart arrythmias, or CAD.

Black Box Warning: High abuse potential [14].

Methylphenidate d, l (Ritalin)

Starting Dose: 5 mg PO in the am and at lunch,

Titration: Increase by 5–10 mg every week.

Max Dose: 60 mg BID.

FDA Approval: ADHD. Narcolepsy.

Common Side Effects: Insomnia, headache, exacerbation of tics, nervousness, irritability, overstimulation, tremor, dizziness, anorexia, dry mouth, nausea.

Uncommon: *Psychotic episodes, seizures, palpitations, priapism, and cardiovascular adverse effects.*

Monitoring: Assess for cardiac disease before initiation. Blood pressure and heart rate should be monitored regularly. Monitor height and weight in children.

Contraindications: Extreme anxiety, motor tics, taking a MAOI, cardiovascular disease, glaucoma, structural cardiac abnormalities, cardiomyopathy, serious heart arrythmias, or CAD.

Black Box Warning: High abuse potential [15].

Methylphenidate d, l (Concerta)

Starting Dose: 18 mg PO daily.

Titration: Increase by 18 mg every week.

Max Dose: 72 mg BID.

FDA Approval: ADHD. Narcolepsy.

Common Side Effects: Insomnia, headache, exacerbation of tics, nervousness, irritability, overstimulation, tremor, dizziness, anorexia, dry mouth, nausea.

Uncommon: *Psychotic episodes, seizures, palpitations, priapism, and cardiovascular adverse effects.*

Monitoring: Assess for cardiac disease before initiation. Blood pressure and heart rate should be monitored regularly. Monitor height and weight in children.

Contraindications: Extreme anxiety, motor tics, taking a MAOI, cardiovascular disease, glaucoma, structural cardiac abnormalities, cardiomyopathy, serious heart arrythmias, or CAD.

Black Box Warning: High abuse potential [16].

Methylphenidate HCL (Jornay PM)

Starting Dose: 20 mg PO nightly.

Titration: Increase by 20 mg every week.

Max Dose: 100 mg daily.

FDA Approval: ADHD in 6 years and older.

Common Side Effects: Insomnia, headache, exacerbation of tics, nervousness, irritability, overstimulation, tremor, dizziness, anorexia, dry mouth, nausea.

Uncommon: *Psychotic episodes, seizures, palpitations, priapism, and cardiovascular adverse effects.*

Monitoring: Assess for cardiac disease before initiation. Blood pressure and heart rate should be monitored regularly. Monitor height and weight in children.

Contraindications: Extreme anxiety, motor tics, taking a MAOI, cardiovascular disease, glaucoma, structural cardiac abnormalities, cardiomyopathy, serious heart arrythmias, or CAD.

Black Box Warning: High abuse potential [17].

Serdexmethylphenidate (Azstarys)

Starting Dose: 39.5 mg/7.8 mg daily.

Titration: Increase to 52.3 mg/10.4 mg daily after 7 days.

Max Dose: 52.3 mg/10.4 mg.

FDA Approval: ADHD for over 6 years of age.

Common Side Effects: Insomnia, headache, exacerbation of tics, nervousness, irritability, overstimulation, tremor, dizziness, anorexia, dry mouth, nausea.

Uncommon: *Psychotic episodes, seizures, palpitations, priapism, and cardiovascular adverse effects.*

Monitoring: Assess for cardiac disease before initiation. Blood pressure and heart rate should be monitored regularly. Monitor height and weight in children.

Contraindications: Extreme anxiety, motor tics, taking a MAOI, cardiovascular disease, glaucoma, structural cardiac abnormalities, cardiomyopathy, serious heart arrythmias, or CAD.

Black Box Warning: High abuse potential [18].

Switching from Methylphenidate to Concerta

5 mg of methylphenidate BID or TID dosing: Start 18 mg Concerta q am

10 mg of methylphenidate BID or TID dosing: Start 36 mg Concerta q am

15 mg of methylphenidate BID or TID dosing: Start 54 mg Concerta q am

References

1. Caplan J, Stern T. Mnemonics in a mnutshell: 32 aids to psychiatric diagnosis. Curr Psychiatr Ther. 2008;7(10):27–33.
2. Moses S, MD. ADHD differential diagnosis; 2022. https://fpnotebook.com/Peds/Neuro/AdhdDfrntlDgns.htmNovartisPharmaceuticalsCorporation.
3. What is ADHD? Centers for Disease Control and Prevention; 2021, January 26. https://www.cdc.gov/ncbddd/adhd/facts.html#Causes.
4. Lovering N. How cognitive behavioral therapy can help with ADHD. Psych Central; 2022, March 28. https://psychcentral.com/adhd/cognitive-behavioral-therapy-for-adhd#cbt-techniques.
5. Eli Lilly and Company. Strattera: highlights of prescribing information; 2002. https://pi.lilly.com/us/strattera-pi.pdf.
6. Concordia Pharmaceuticals. Kapvay: highlights of prescribing information; 2022. https://www.accessdata.fda.gov/drugsatfda_docs/label/2020/022331s021lbl.pdf.
7. Shire US Inc. Guanfacine: highlights of prescribing information; 2017. https://www.accessdata.fda.gov/drugsatfda_docs/label/2019/022037s018lbl.pdf.
8. Supernus Pharmaceuticals Inc. Qelbree: highlights of prescribing information; 2022. https://www.supernus.com/sites/default/files/Qelbree-Prescribing-Info.pdf.

9. Catalent Pharma Solutions. Dexedrine: prescribing information; 2023. https://www.accessdata.fda.gov/drugsatfda_docs/label/2023/017078s055lbl.pdf.
10. DSM Pharmaceuticals Inc. Adderall: medication guide; 2007. https://www.accessdata.fda.gov/drugsatfda_docs/label/2007/011522s040lbl.pdf.
11. Takeda Pharmaceutical Company. Adderall XR: highlights of prescribing information; 2019. https://www.accessdata.fda.gov/drugsatfda_docs/label/2019/021303s034lbl.pdf..
12. Takeda Pharmaceutical Company. Vyvanse: highlights of prescribing information; 2021. https://www.accessdata.fda.gov/drugsatfda_docs/label/2021/021977s046,208510s003lbl.pdf.
13. Novartis Pharmaceuticals Corporation. Focalin: prescribing information; 2012. https://www.accessdata.fda.gov/drugsatfda_docs/label/2012/021278s015lbl.pdf.
14. Focalin XR. Prescribing information; 2004. https://www.accessdata.fda.gov/drugsatfda_docs/label/2005/021802lbl.pdf.
15. Novartis Pharmaceuticals Corporation. Ritalin: prescribing information; 2007. https://www.accessdata.fda.gov/drugsatfda_docs/label/2007/010187s069,018029s040,021284s011lbl.pdf.
16. Janssen Pharmaceuticals. Concerta: highlights of prescribing information; 2013. https://www.accessdata.fda.gov/drugsatfda_docs/label/2021/021121s044lbl.pdf.
17. Ironshore Pharmaceuticals. Jornay: highlights of prescribing information; 2023. https://ironshorepharma.com/wpcontent/uploads/2023/10/JORNAY_PM_Label.pdf#page=1.
18. Corium LLC. Azstarys: highlights of prescribing information; 2023. https://corium.com/products/AZSTARYS/AZSTARYS_PI_ENGLISH_US.pdf.

Bipolar Disorder

4

Contents

B. Floyd, T. Kane, *The Clinician's Guide to Common Psychiatric Disorders*, https://doi.org/10.1007/978-3-031-67958-2_4

Bipolar Disorder

Bipolar disorder is a mood disorder characterized by extreme mood swings and/or emotional highs (Mania/Hypomania) and lows (Depression). Depressive symptoms are hallmarked by persistent feelings of sadness, loss of interest, and/or anhedonia (lack of pleasure). (Hypo)mania symptoms are hallmarked by unusually high amounts of energy, decreased need for sleep, grandiosity, and sometimes irritability. The patient can also have both depressive and hypomanic symptoms at the same time, known as mixed mood.

Diagnosing and Monitoring

Mnemonic: Depressed mood and 5 or more symptoms lasting for more than 2 weeks.

SIGE-CAPS: Depressed mood and 5 or more: **S**uicidal thoughts, **I**nterest decreased, **G**uilt, **E**nergy decreased, **C**oncentration decreased, **A**ppetite disturbance, **P**sychomotor agitation/retardation, **S**leep disturbances [1].

Mnemonic: 3 or more, 4 if only irritable mood for 4+ days for hypomania, more than 7 days for mania.

DIGFAST: **D**istractibility, **I**nsomnia, **G**randiosity, **F**light of ideas, **A**ctivities (increased), **S**peech, **T**houghtlessness (risk taking behavior) [1].

Bipolar diagnosis is made if a patient has had a major depressive episode and one hypomanic/manic episode. The biggest risk factor of bipolar is first-degree relative with bipolar disorder.

DSM-5-TR

According to the DSM-5-TR, to have a diagnosis of bipolar disorder, the patient must have at least one episode of (hypo)mania and at least one episode of major depressive disorder. The difference between Bipolar 1 and Bipolar II is the severity of the (hypo)manic episode. A manic episode must last for at least 7 days and at least 4 days for a hypomanic episode. If the mania is so severe that it warrants hospitalization, it is more than likely a Bipolar 1 diagnosis.

(Hypo)mania is defined as a persistently elevated mood that is an obvious change from baseline. It can also include an irritable mood and increased energy lasting for 1 week for mania and 4 days for hypomania. There will also be at least three of the following symptoms, four if the mood is irritable [2, p. 140]:

1. Grandiosity.
2. Decreased need for sleep
3. Pressured speech/more talkative
4. Flight of ideas or mind racing
5. Easily distracted
6. Increase in goal-directed activity or psychomotor agitation
7. High risk/impulsive behaviors (shopping sprees, excessive alcohol/substance abuse, sexual indiscretions, etc.)

The mood is severe enough to cause impairment in every day life. The mood is not attributable to a physiological effect, drug, or better explained by another mental illness (Schizoaffective).

Major Depressive Disorder

The DSM-5-TR is used to diagnose Major Depressive Disorder. In order to have an MDD diagnoses, you must have at least one of the first two symptoms listed and a total of five symptoms for more than a 2-week period. These symptoms are [2, p. 141] as follows:

- **Depressed mood**
- **Decreased interest/pleasure** in things you used to find interesting/pleasurable
- Decrease/increase in appetite nearly every day
- Insomnia/hypersomnia
- Psychomotor agitation/retardation
- Energy loss
- Decreased concentration
- Recurrent thoughts of death or suicide without a plan

Like all diagnoses in the DSM-5-TR, the illness should cause significant distress in the individual's life. Also, it cannot better be explained by a medical condition, substance, or other mental health disorder that would better explain the symptoms. There also must have never been a (hypo)manic episode. For a more comprehensive review, see the DSM-5-TR.

Bipolar 1 Versus Bipolar 2

Bipolar 1 versus Bipolar 2 is determined by the severity of the (hypo)manic episode. If the patient meets criteria for a hypomanic episode and has never experienced a manic episode, they would be Bipolar 2. If a patient meets criteria for a manic episode and there is significant dysfunction/need for hospitalization, they would be Bipolar 1.

It is important to note that Bipolar 2 is not just a mild form of Bipolar 1 but is a distinct diagnosis. Patients with Bipolar 2 will not have symptoms severe enough to be classified as manic but they will spend significantly more time in a depressed state.

Hypomania

- Lasts at least 4 consecutive days.
- Typically, not severe enough to significantly affect social or work/school functioning.
- Usually no need for hospitalization. If hospitalization is necessary, it is not hypomania.

Mania

- Lasts at least 7 consecutive days
- Causes severe impact on social or work/school functioning
- May possibly need hospitalization for stabilization [3]

Differential Diagnosis: Anxiety disorders, hyperthyroidism, neurosyphilis, ADHD, PTSD, schizoaffective disorder, schizophrenia, and SAD.

Risk Factors: First-degree relative with bipolar, periods of high stress, and drug or alcohol abuse.

Labs to Consider: Complete blood count (CBC), complete metabolic panel (CMP) thyroid functioning tests, B12 levels, vitamin D, and folate levels. Urine drug screen if warranted. If the patient reports snoring, excessive daytime sleepiness, or apnea, consider sleep study.

Screening Scales

PHQ-9: It is a nine question, self-administered diagnostic tool that rates the severity of depression based on the last 2 weeks. It takes less than 3 min to complete and is the most popular depression screener.

HAM-D: It has 21 questions with only 17 being scored for severity of depression. It is clinician administered and more in depth while also being more time consuming than PHQ-9. It takes about 15 min to complete.

HAM-D6: It is an abbreviated six question, self-administered test. It can be completed in less than 3 min.

Beck Depression Inventory: It consists of 21 questions about how the patient has been feeling in the last week. It helps with diagnosis but also with severity of illness.

Geriatric Depression Scale: Long form is 30 questions, while short form is 15. It is used with older adults mostly in acute, long-term, and community settings.

Screening Scales: Mania

***Altman Self-Rating Mania Scale*: It is a 5**-item self-reported diagnostic scale which can be used to assess the presence and severity manic and hypomanic symptoms.

***CARS-M*: It is a** 15-item, clinician-rated scale used to assess symptoms of mania and psychosis experienced by a patient over the last 7 days.

Young Mania Rating Scale: It is an 11-item multiple choice diagnostic questionnaire that measures the presence and severity of mania and associated symptoms.

***Rapid Mood Screener (RMS)*: It is a** six question screening tool that should take less than 2 min to complete. Four out of six positives suggests a need for further evaluation for Bipolar 1. It has a sensitivity and specificity of 88% and 80%.

Treatment

First-line treatment for bipolar disorder is pharmacotherapy. Psychotherapy is recommended based on availability of therapies and patient need. Not all patients with bipolar will need psychotherapy. Therapy should be aimed at psychoeducation on diagnosis, adhering to treatment, and developing healthy lifestyle choices such as proper diet, exercise, and avoiding drugs and alcohol as this can exacerbate the symptoms of bipolar. For patients that are psychotic, suicidal, or catatonic, electroconvulsive therapy (ECT) is a viable option.

Non-pharmacologic Interventions

Cognitive Behavioral Therapy (CBT): It is a type of therapy that focuses on changing one's thoughts and behaviors to improve mood and functioning. It is a short-term, collaborative, goal-oriented therapy where the therapist helps the client identify negative thought patterns and behaviors. Together they develop ways to reconceptualize these thoughts and behaviors into something more positive. It is the most popular type of therapy.

Interpersonal Therapy (IPT): It is a type of therapy that focuses on interpersonal relationships and social interactions that can have an impact on a patient's mental health. The therapist will help identify problem areas in the patient's relationships and outline ways to address the difficulties which will in turn help alleviate depressive symptoms.

Electroconvulsive Therapy (ECT)

Background: ECT has been in use since the 1920s but is being used less frequently due to the stigma surrounding it. ECT is the most efficacious treatment for bipolar that is available at this time. It also is the most invasive of all treatment options.

How It Works: ECT involves a very complex mechanism of action that is not completely understood. Inducing a seizure seems to "reset" the brain and cause the release of chemicals related to mood regulation, quickly alleviating depressive, catatonic, and psychotic symptoms.

Patient Experience: The patient will be placed on a stretcher in the procedure room. An IV will be inserted and the patient will have an oxygen mask placed. The patient will then be told to take deep breaths and an anesthetic will be given. The patient will fall asleep and the provider will use an electrode to deliver an electrical current to elicit a seizure. The patient will be unaware that anything has happened and will wake up in 5–10 min. They will be sleepy and possibly confused. They will be monitored in recovery for around 30 min and then released home. The patient is unable to drive for the day.

Pharmacologic Interventions

Treatments Based on Mood State

Bipolar: Depressed	Caplyta, Latuda, Seroquel/XR, and Symbyax
Bipolar: Manic	Abilify, Depakote, Equetro, Lithium, Saphris, Seroquel/XR, Vraylar, Zyprexa
Bipolar: Mixed Mood State	Abilify, Depakote, Equetro, Lithium, Saphris, Vraylar, Zyprexa
Bipolar: Maintenance	Abilify, Depakote, Lamictal, Lithium, Risperdal, Saphris, Seroquel, Zyprexa
Bipolar 2	Seroquel XR and Caplyta

****Before starting any atypical antipsychotic, you should weigh all patients and track BMI during treatment. Also document waist circumference, blood pressure, fasting plasma glucose, and fasting lipid profile.****

One should be mindful of patients developing metabolic syndrome which would be three or more of the following:

1. Waistline of 40 in. for men or 35 in. for women
2. Blood pressure above 130/85
3. Triglyceride level above 150
4. Fasting blood glucose greater than 100
5. HDL less than 40 in men or 50 in women [4]

First-Line Medications

Mood Stabilizers

Carbamazepine (Equetro)

Starting Dose: 200 mg PO twice daily.

Titration: Increase by 200 mg PO daily every week.

Max Dose: 1200 mg/day.

FDA Approval: Acute mania (bipolar), mixed mania (bipolar), partial seizures with complex symptomatology, generalized tonic-clonic seizures, mixed seizure patterns, trigeminal neuralgia pain.

Common Side Effects: Rash, benign leukopenia, GI upset, dry mouth, blurred vision, sedation, dizziness, unsteadiness, and confusion.

Rare: *Aplastic anemia, agranulocytosis, severe dermatologic reactions such as SJS and purpura, anaphylaxis, induction of psychosis or mania, SIADH, and activation of suicidal ideation and behavior.*

Monitoring: Initiation: CBC, CMP, and thyroid. During treatment: CBC q for 2–4 weeks for 2 months and then q for 3–6 months. CMP and thyroid q for 6–12 months.

Contraindications: History of bone marrow suppression, allergy to carbamazepine, proven allergy to any tricyclic compound, and positive test for HLA-B*1502 allele.

Black Box Warning: Serious dermatologic reactions (toxic epidermal necrolysis and Stevens-Johnson syndrome) and aplastic anemia/agranulocytosis [5].

Divalproex (Depakote ER)

Starting Dose: Mania: 25 mg/kg/day.

Titration: 10–20 mg/kg/day.

Max Dose: 60 mg/kg/day.

FDA Approval: Acute mania and mixed episodes, seizures, migraine prophylaxis, bipolar maintenance.

Common Side Effects: Sedation, tremor, dizziness, abdominal pain, N/V/D, reduced appetite, constipation, heart burn, weight gain, ataxia, asthenia, headache, *tachycardia/bradycardia*.

Rare: *Hepatotoxicity, pancreatitis, DRESS, activation of suicidal ideation.*

Monitoring: CBC, CMP at baseline. LFT frequently. If tired or confused, draw ammonia.

Contraindications: Pancreatitis, severe liver disease, urea cycle disorder.

Pearls: Do not use with women with PCOS. Only use half dose if adding Lamictal (Blue starter pack).

Black Box Warning: Use may result to increased risk of pancreatitis and liver failure [6].

Lamotrigine (Lamictal) (Goal Is 150–250 mg)

Starting Dose: 25 mg PO daily.

Titration: Increase by 25 mg every 2 weeks.

Max Dose: 400 mg PO daily and higher have been used.

FDA Approval: Maintenance treatment of Bipolar 1, partial seizures, and tonic/clonic seizures.

Common Side Effects: Benign rash, blurred vision, dizziness, ataxia, sedation, headache, tremor, insomnia, poor coordination, and fatigue.

Rare: *Serious rash, Stevens-Johnson syndrome, blood dyscrasias, aseptic meningitis, hemophagocytic lymphohistiocytosis.*

Monitoring: Creatinine at baseline. Eye exam for prolonged treatment. Assess for depression and SI.

Pearls: If adding Depakote, only use half the dose instead of full Depakote dose. Start 125 mg PO QHS. With slow titration, you may need atypical such as Vraylar. It can take months for proper titration.

Black Box Warning: Use may result to life-threatening serious rashes including Stevens-Johnson syndrome, toxic epidermal necrolysis, and/or rash-related death [7].

Lithium (It Is Best for Mania and Depression as well as Suicidality. It Helps Preserve Brain Size)

Starting Dose: 300 mg PO TID.

Titration: Increase by 300 mg/day every 3 days.

Max Dose: 1800 mg PO daily.

FDA Approval: Manic episodes, acute mania/mixed mania, maintenance treatment for manic-depressive patients with history of mania, and bipolar maintenance.

Common Side Effects: Ataxia, dysarthria, delirium, tremor, memory problems, polyura, polydipsia, diarrhea, nausea, weight gain, goiter, hypothyroidism, acne, rash, alopecia, metallic taste, leukocytosis, *renal impairment, nephrogenic diabetes insipidus, arrythmia, sick sinus syndrome, hypotension.*

Monitoring: CBC, CMP, TSH baseline, 1 month after treatment and then q for 6 months. Drug levels twice weekly until stable then q for 2 months until chronic steady dose. Parathyroid for low calcium. Lithium level goals: Acute treatment: 1.0–1.5 mEq/L, Chronic treatment: 0.6–1.2 mEq/L.

Pearls: Decreased risk of suicidality.

Contraindications: Severe kidney disease, severe cardiovascular disease, Brugada syndrome, severe dehydration, or sodium depletion.

Black Box Warning: Lithium toxicity is closely related to lithium blood levels and can occur at doses close to therapeutic levels [8].

Second-Generation Antipsychotics

Aripiprazole (Abilify)

Starting Dose: Mania: 5–10 mg PO daily.

Titration: Increase by 5 mg PO daily every week.

Max Dose: 30 mg PO daily.

FDA Approval: Depression adjunct, schizophrenia, bipolar maintenance, autism-related irritability in children ages 6–17, Tourette's disorder in children ages 6–18, acute agitation associated with schizophrenia and bipolar.

Common Side Effects: Dizziness, insomnia, akathisia, activation, nausea, vomiting, headache, orthostatic hypotension, tardive dyskinesia.

Rare: Impulse control problems (gambling), *hyperglycemia, neuroleptic malignant syndrome, seizures.*

Monitoring: PHQ-9, BMI every 3 months, lipid panel, and A1c annually. Waist circumference, blood pressure, fasting plasma glucose, and fasting lipid profile prior to start, within 3 months, and then annually. AIMS score every 3–6 months.

Pearl: Injectable form available.

Black Box Warning: Elderly dementia patients who take Abilify have a higher risk of death. Use may increase suicidal thoughts in children, adolescents, and young adults [9].

Asenapine (Saphris)

Starting Dose: Mania: 10 mg sublingual BID (20 mg/day).

Titration: May reduce to 5 mg sublingual BID (10 mg/day) if adverse effects.

Max Dose: 20 mg/day.

FDA Approval: Schizophrenia, mania/mixed mania, and bipolar maintenance.

Common Side Effects: Increased risk for diabetes and dyslipidemia, dizziness, sedation, dry mouth, constipation, weight gain, edema, musculoskeletal pain, orthostatic hypotension, tardive dyskinesia.

Rare: *Type-1 hypersensitivity reactions, hyperglycemia (ketoacidosis), NMS.*

Monitoring: PHQ-9, BMI every 3 months, lipid panel, and A1c annually. Waist circumference, blood pressure, fasting plasma glucose, and fasting lipid profile prior to start, within 3 months, and then annually. AIMS score every 3–6 months.

Black Box Warning: Elderly dementia patients who take Saphris have a higher risk of death. Use may increase suicidal thoughts in children, adolescents, and young adults (24 and younger) [10].

Cariprazine (Vraylar)

Starting Dose: 1.5 mg po daily.

Titration: Mania: Increase to 3 mg PO daily on day 2.
Depression: Increase to 3 mg PO daily on day 15.

Max Dose: 6 mg. Recommended range 3–6 mg.

FDA Approval: Schizophrenia acute and maintenance, acute mania/mixed mood, Bipolar 1 (depression), MDD adjunct.

Common Side Effects: Akathisia, EPS, restlessness, GI distress, sedation, tardive dyskinesia.

Rare: *Hyperglycemia, neuroleptic malignant syndrome, and seizures.*

Monitoring: PHQ-9, BMI every 3 months, lipid panel, and A1c annually. Waist circumference, blood pressure, fasting plasma glucose, and fasting lipid profile prior to start, within 3 months, and then annually. AIMS score every 3–6 months.

Caveats: Side effects may develop weeks later due to long half-life.

Black Box Warning: Elderly dementia patients who take Abilify have a higher risk of death. Use may increase suicidal thoughts in children, adolescents, and young adults [11].

Lumateperone (Caplyta)

Starting Dose: 42 mg.

Titration: None needed.

Max 42 mg.

FDA Approval: Schizophrenia, bipolar depression.

Common Side Effects: Sedation, nausea, dry mouth, tardive dyskinesia.

Uncommon: *Hyperglycemia, neuroleptic malignant syndrome, stroke, orthostatic hypotension, low white blood cell count,* and *seizures.*

Monitoring: BMI monthly × 3 months then every 3 months. Blood pressure, fasting plasma glucose, fasting lipid panel within 3 months and then monthly. More often if at risk for metabolic syndrome. AIMS score every 3–6 months.

Caveats: It is not known for metabolic side effects. New dosage forms are available: 10 mg, 21 mg, and 42 mg.

Black Box Warning: Elderly dementia patients who take Abilify have a higher risk of death. Use may increase suicidal thoughts in children, adolescents, and young adults [12].

Lurasidone (Latuda)

Starting Dose: 20 mg PO daily with largest meal.

Titration: Increase by 5–10 mg PO daily every week.

Max Dose: 120 mg PO daily.

FDA Approval: Schizophrenia, bipolar depression.

Common Side Effects: Sedation, akathisia, nausea, hyperprolactinemia, increased risk of diabetes and dyslipidemia, tardive dyskinesia.

Rare: *Tachycardia/first-degree AV block, hyperglycemia (ketoacidosis), NMS, seizures.*

Monitoring: BMI monthly × 3 months then every 3 months. Blood pressure, fasting plasma glucose, fasting lipid panel within 3 months and then monthly. More often if at risk for metabolic syndrome. AIMS score every 3–6 months.

Caveats: Give with >350 calories. Used in depressed state, watch for s/s of mania.

Contraindications: Taking a strong CYP 3A4 inhibitor/inducer (ketoconazole, rifampin), history of angioedema.

Black Box Warning: Elderly dementia patients who take Abilify have a higher risk of death. Use may increase suicidal thoughts in children, adolescents, and young adults [13].

Olanzapine (Zyprexa)

Starting Dose: 5–10 mg PO nightly.
Titration: 5 mg PO nightly every week.
Max Dose: 20 mg/day.
FDA Approval: Treatment-resistant depression, schizophrenia, bipolar maintenance, bipolar depression.
Common Side Effects: Increased risk for diabetes and dyslipidemia, dizziness, sedation, dry mouth, constipation, weight gain, edema, musculoskeletal pain, orthostatic hypotension, tardive dyskinesia.
Rare: *DRESS*, *hyperglycemia (ketoacidosis)*, *NMS*, *seizures*.
Monitoring: GAD-7, BMI every 3 months, lipid panel, and A1c annually. Waist circumference, blood pressure, fasting plasma glucose, and fasting lipid profile prior to start, within 3 months, and then annually. AIMS score every 3–6 months.
Contraindications: Risk of angle-closure glaucoma, unstable cardiac condition.
Black Box Warning: Elderly dementia patients who take Zyprexa have a higher risk of death. Use may increase suicidal thoughts in children, adolescents, and young adults (24 and younger) [14].

Olanzapine-Fluoxetine (Symbyax)

Starting Dose: 6 mg/25 mg mg PO daily.
Titration: Increase by 3 mg of olanzapine or 25 mg of fluoxetine.
Max Dose: 18 mg/75 mg mg PO daily.
FDA Approval: Treatment-resistant depression, schizophrenia, bipolar maintenance, bipolar depression.
Common Side Effects: Increased risk of diabetes and dyslipidemia, dizziness, sedation, dry mouth, constipation, weight gain, edema, musculoskeletal pain, orthostatic hypotension, tardive dyskinesia.
Rare: *DRESS, hyperglycemia, neuroleptic malignant syndrome, seizures.*

Monitoring: PHQ-9, BMI every 3 months, lipid panel, and A1c annually. Waist circumference, blood pressure, fasting plasma glucose, and fasting lipid profile prior to start, within 3 months, and then annually. AIMS score every 3–6 months.

Contraindications: Known risk of angle-closure glaucoma or unstable cardiac condition.

Black Box Warning: Elderly dementia patients who take Symbyax have a higher risk of death. Use may increase suicidal thoughts in children, adolescents, and young adults (24 and younger) [15].

Quetiapine (Seroquel)

Starting Dose: 50 mg PO BID.

Titration: 100 mg/day. Once at 400 mg/day, it may increase by 200 mg/day.

Max Dose: 800 mg PO daily.

FDA Approval: MDD, bipolar depression, bipolar maintenance, schizophrenia.

Common Side Effects: GI upset, sexual dysfunction, insomnia, agitation, sedation, dizziness, urinary retention, headache, weight loss, myalgia, sweating, anorexia, hypertension, and nausea better in 3–5 days.

Rare: *Neuroleptic malignant syndrome, hyperglycemia, and seizures.*

Monitoring: PHQ-9, BMI every 3 months, lipid panel, and A1c annually. Waist circumference, blood pressure, fasting plasma glucose, and fasting lipid profile prior to start, within 3 months, and then annually. AIMS score every 3–6 months.

Pearl: Known for sedating properties, it could be a useful insomnia adjunct in doses up to 100 mg.

Black Box Warning: Elderly dementia patients who take Seroquel have a higher risk of death. Use may increase suicidal thoughts in children, adolescents, and young adults (24 and younger) [16, 17].

Quetiapine XR (Seroquel XR)

Starting Dose: Mania: 300 mg PO nightly.
Bipolar Depression: 150 mg PO nightly.

Titration: Mania: It may increase by 300 mg PO nightly each day.
Bipolar Depression: Titrate as needed to reach 300 mg/night by day 4.

Max Dose: Usually 800 mg PO daily for bipolar.

FDA Approval: MDD, bipolar depression, bipolar maintenance, schizophrenia.

Common Side Effects: GI upset, sexual dysfunction, insomnia, agitation, sedation, dizziness, urinary retention, headache, weight loss, myalgia, sweating, anorexia, hypertension, and nausea better in 3–5 days.

Rare: *Neuroleptic malignant syndrome, hyperglycemia, and seizures.*

Monitoring: PHQ-9, BMI every 3 months, lipid panel, and A1c annually. Waist circumference, blood pressure, fasting plasma glucose, and fasting lipid profile prior to start, within 3 months and then annually. AIMS score every 3–6 months.

Black Box Warning: Elderly dementia patients who take Seroquel have a higher risk of death. Use may increase suicidal thoughts in children, adolescents, and young adults (24 and younger) [16, 17].

Risperidone (Risperdal)

Starting Dose: 0.5 mg PO BID (1 mg/day).

Titration: Increase by 1 mg/day, every day.

Max Dose: 16 mg/day.

FDA Approval: Schizophrenia, acute mania/mixed mania, autism-related irritability in children, and bipolar maintenance.

Common Side Effects: Increased risk for diabetes and dyslipidemia, drug-induced parkinsonism, hyperprolactinemia, dizziness, insomnia, anxiety, sedation, GI distress, weight gain, sexual dysfunction, tardive dyskinesia, and orthostatic hypotension.

Uncommon/Rare: *Hyperglycemia, neuroleptic malignant syndrome, seizures.*

Monitoring: PHQ-9, BMI every 3 months, lipid panel, and A1c annually. Waist circumference, blood pressure, fasting plasma glucose, and fasting lipid profile prior to start, within 3 months and then annually. AIMS score every 3–6 months.

Black Box Warning: Elderly dementia patients who take Zyprexa have a higher risk of death. Use may increase suicidal thoughts in children, adolescents, and young adults (24 and younger) [18].

Cyclothymic Disorder

Cyclothymic disorder is a relatively rare persistent mood disorder (greater than 2 years by definition) that is defined by cycling of emotional highs and lows. The highs are not extreme enough to qualify for hypomania, and the depressive symptoms are not low enough to qualify for major depressive disorder. However, it is important to seek treatment because there is an increased risk of developing bipolar later in life.

Diagnosing and Monitoring

DSM-5-TR

Cyclothymic disorder is a mood disorder that has hypomanic and depressive symptoms, but the patient does not reach full criteria for the diagnosis. If the patient has several hypomanic symptoms and several depressive symptoms for the past 2 years, they may be experiencing cyclothymia. Symptoms must be present for at least half of the time over the 2-year period, and the patient cannot be without symptoms for more than 2 months. The illness is nor attributable to another physiological cause, drug, or better explained by another mental illness (Schizoaffective). For a more comprehensive review, see the DSM-5-TR [2, p. 159].

Differential Diagnosis: MDD, Bipolar 2, generalized anxiety disorder, personality disorders, neurodevelopmental disorders, and medical causes (endocrine disorders, electrolyte abnormalities, infection, steroids, withdrawal from drugs of abuse).

Risk Factors: First-degree relative with bipolar, periods of high stress, and drug or alcohol abuse.

Labs to Consider: Complete blood count (CBC), complete metabolic panel (CMP) thyroid functioning tests, B12 levels, vitamin D, and folate levels. Urine drug screen if warranted. If the patient reports snoring, excessive daytime sleepiness, or apnea, consider sleep study.

Screening Scales

PHQ-9: It is a 9-question, self-administered diagnostic tool that rates the severity of depression based on the last 2 weeks. It takes less than 3 min to complete and is the most popular depression screener.

HAM-D: It has 21 questions with only 17 being scored for severity of depression. It is clinician administered and more in depth while also being more time consuming than PHQ-9. It takes about 15 min to complete.

HAM-D6: It is an abbreviated 6-question, self-administered test. It can be completed in less than 3 min.

Beck Depression Inventory: It consists of 21 questions about how the patient has been feeling in the last week. It helps with diagnosis but also with severity of illness.

Geriatric Depression Scale: Long form is 30 questions while short form is 15. It is used with older adults mostly in acute, long-term, and community settings.

Screening Scales: Mania

***Altman Self-Rating Mania Scale*: It is a** 5-item self-reported diagnostic scale which can be used to assess the presence and severity manic and hypomanic symptoms.

***CARS-M*: It is a** 15-item, clinician-rated scale used to assess symptoms of mania and psychosis experienced by a patient over the last 7 days.

Young Mania Rating Scale: It is an 11-item multiple choice diagnostic questionnaire that measures the presence and severity of mania and associated symptoms.

***Rapid Mood Screener (RMS)*: It is a** 6-question screening tool that should take less than 2 min to complete. 4 out of 6 positive suggests the need for further evaluation for Bipolar 1. It has a sensitivity and specificity of 88% and 80%.

Treatment

There is no FDA-approved medication for cyclothymic disorder. However, the patient should be treated to mitigate symptoms and lessen the chance of poor prognosis. First-line medications are typically mood stabilizers such as Depakote, Lithium, or Lamictal. If anxiety is high, Depakote may be the better choice, and if it is a predominant anxious/depressed type, then Lamictal maybe a good choice. Second-generation antipsychotics may also be used. However, it is best to avoid antidepressants without an effective mood stabilizer in place as this could exacerbate symptoms. First-line psychotherapy is a cognitive behavioral therapy. Therapy should be aimed at affective dysregulation, while psychoeducation should include medication adherence, acceptance of diagnosis, self-care, regular exercise, and well-balanced diet.

References

1. Caplan J, Stern T. Mnemonics in a mnutshell: 32 aids to psychiatric diagnosis. Curr Psychiatr Ther. 2008;7(10):27–33.
2. American Psychiatric Association. Mood disorders. In: Diagnostic and statistical manual of mental disorders (5th-TR). Washington, DC: American Psychiatric Association; 2022.
3. Hypomania. Cleveland Clinic; 2024. https://my.clevelandclinic.org/health/diseases/21774-hypomania.

4. Driggins SN, Muhammad KR. A population at risk: a metabolic syndrome study among African American Students at a Historically Black College and University. Athens J Health Med Sci. 2019;6(4):231–42. https://doi.org/10.30958/ajhms.6-4-3.
5. Validus Pharmaceuticals LLC. Equetro: highlights of prescribing information; 2021. https://equetro.com/static/pdf/equetro-prescribing-info.pdf.
6. AbbVie. Depakote ER: highlights of prescribing information; 2017. https://www.accessdata.fda.gov/drugsatfda_docs/label/2018/021168s038lbl.pdf.
7. GlaxoSmithKline. Lamictal: highlights of prescribing information; 2010. https://www.accessdata.fda.gov/drugsatfda_docs/label/2010/020241s043s044,020764s036s037,022251s005s006lbl.pdf.
8. West-Ward Pharmaceuticals. Lithium: highlights of prescribing information; 2018. https://www.accessdata.fda.gov/drugsatfda_docs/label/2018/017812s033,018421s032,018558s027lbl.pdf.
9. Otsuka American Pharmaceutical, Inc. Abilify: highlights of prescribing information; 2022. https://www.otsuka-us.com/sites/g/files/qhldwo7626/files/media/static/Abilify-PI.pdf.
10. Merck S, Dohme BV. Saphris: highlights of prescribing information; 2017. https://www.accessdata.fda.gov/drugsatfda_docs/label/2017/022117s020s021lbl.pdf.
11. Forest Laboratories Holdings Ltd. Vraylar: highlights of prescribing information; 2022. https://www.rxabbvie.com/pdf/vraylar_pi.pdf.
12. Intracellular Therapies. Caplyta: highlights of prescribing information; 2023. https://www.intracellulartherapies.com/docs/caplyta_pi.pdf.
13. Sunovion Pharmaceuticals Inc. Latuda: highlights of prescribing information; 2013. https://www.accessdata.fda.gov/drugsatfda_docs/label/2013/200603lbls10s11.pdf.
14. Eli Lilly and Company. Zyprexa: highlights of prescribing information; 2021. https://pi.lilly.com/us/zyprexa-pi.pdf
15. Eli Lilly and Company. Symbyax: Highlights of Prescribing Information; 2023. https://pi.lilly.com/us/symbyax-pi.pdf
16. AstraZeneca Pharmaceuticals LP. Seroquel: highlights of prescribing information; 2009. https://www.accessdata.fda.gov/drugsatfda_docs/label/2009/020639s045s046lbl.pdf.
17. AstraZeneca Pharmaceuticals LP. Seroquel XR: highlights of prescribing information; 2009. https://www.accessdata.fda.gov/drugsatfda_docs/label/2009/022047s011s016s017s019s022lbl.pdf.
18. Janssen Pharmaceutical Companies. Risperdal: highlights of prescribing information; 2007. https://www.accessdata.fda.gov/drugsatfda_docs/label/2019/020272s082,020588s070,021444s056lbl.pdf.

Obsessive Compulsive Disorder (OCD)

5

Contents

Obsessive Compulsive Disorder

Obsessive-compulsive disorder (OCD) is a mental health disorder hallmarked by unwanted, uncontrollable, and recurring thoughts or obsessions. Compulsions are repetitive behaviors a person feels the urge to do, often to lessen the anxiety related to their obsessions. The obsessions/compulsions are time consuming and have a significant impact on day to day life. Common obsessions are fear of contamination, extreme worrying about cleanliness or symmetry, violent or aggressive imagery, and repetitive doubts or questions. Common compulsions include excessive hand washing, counting, checking locks or appliances, tapping, or repeating certain phrases.

B. Floyd, T. Kane, *The Clinician's Guide to Common Psychiatric Disorders*, https://doi.org/10.1007/978-3-031-67958-2_5

Diagnosing and Monitoring

Mnemonic

MURDER: **M**ind (symptoms are in their mind), **U**npleasant thoughts, **R**esist (want to and try to resist thoughts), **D**ispleasure of the obsession, **E**go-dystonic, **R**epetitive thoughts [1].

DSM-5-TR

The DSM-5-TR lists OCD as the presence of either a compulsion or obsession. An obsession is defined as [2, p. 265]:

> Recurrent and persistent thoughts, urges, or images that are experienced, at some time during the disturbance, as intrusive and unwanted, and that in the most individuals cause marked anxiety or distress.
>
> AND
>
> The individual attempts to ignore or suppress such thoughts, urges, or images, or to neutralize them with some other thought or action (i.e., by performing a compulsion).

Compulsions are defined by [2, p. 265]:

> Repetitive behaviors (e.g., hand washing, ordering, checking) or mental acts (e.g., praying, counting, repeating words silently) that the individual feels drive to perform in response to an obsession or according to rules that must be applied rigidly
>
> AND
>
> The behaviors or mental acts are aimed at preventing or reducing anxiety or distress, or preventing some dreaded event or situation; however, these behaviors or mental acts are not connected in a realistic way with what they are designed to neutralize or prevent, or are clearly excessive.

The obsessions/compulsions are not better explained by another mental illness, drug, or physiological effect. Finally, the obsessions/compulsions are time consuming, consuming at least 1 h out of the day.

Differential Diagnosis: Pediatric autoimmune neuropsychiatric disorders associated with streptococcal infections (PANDAS), ruminations with MDD, eating disorder, trichotillomania, obsessive-compulsive personality disorder, tic/stereotypic movement disorder, anxiety disorders, PTSD, hyperthyroidism, and sleep/wake disorders.

Risk Factors: First-degree relative with OCD, first-degree relative with Tourette's syndrome, stressful life events, and comorbid psychiatric diagnoses.

Labs to Consider: Nonspecific to OCD.

Screening Scales

Obsessive Compulsive Inventory: Self-report questionnaire that measures the severity of OCD symptoms. It consists of 42 questions that assess the level of distress among common OCD behaviors such as handwashing, checking, and hoarding. Symptoms are rated from 0 (none) to 4 (extreme). This is not a diagnostic tool and may be used to evaluate level of severity.

Yale-Brown Obsessive-Compulsive Scale: Considered the "gold standard" assessment tool for OCD. The scale consists of 54 common obsessions and compulsions among common themes or behavioral expressions that are rated in severity starting at 0 (none) to 4 (extreme). Scores are combined with obsessive and compulsive symptom severity scores to come to a total OCD severity score.

Treatment

First-line treatment for OCD is cognitive behavioral therapy using exposure and response prevention (CBT/ERP). It is the gold standard of OCD treatment and you should refer to an appropriate therapist. When symptoms are severe or if the patient opts out of therapy and medications are needed, SSRIs are first-line medications. SSRIs will typically be used at higher doses than doses used for depression. Titrate the same way for OCD that would be done for MDD.

Non-pharmacologic Interventions

Cognitive behavioral therapy using exposure and response prevention (CBT/ERP): This is a type of therapy that exposes a patient to a stimulus, in a controlled environment, that would normally elicit a maladaptive response (compulsion) in the patient. In time, the goal is for the patient to develop appropriate responses to the stimuli that will supersede the compulsion impulse when the patient encounters the stimulus in the future.

Pharmacological Interventions

The following chart shows typical dosage ranges of antidepressants when used to treat OCD. The bolded drugs are FDA approved:

Maximum Dosage of SSRIs for OCD

Escitalopram/Lexapro	60 mg/day
Fluoxetine/Prozac	120 mg/day
Fluvoxamine/Luvox	400 mg/day
Paroxetine/Paxil	100 mg/day
Sertraline/Zoloft	400 mg/day

Jiao et al. [3]

Clomipramine (Anafranil)

Starting Dose: 25 mg PO daily.

Titration: Increase (as tolerated) to get to 100 mg po daily at week 2.

Max Dose: 250 mg PO daily.

FDA Approval: Obsessive compulsive disorder.

Common Side Effects: Blurred vision, constipation, dry mouth, weight gain, dizziness, sedation, fatigue, rash, GI upset, sexual dysfunction, sweating, insomnia, agitation, headache, nausea better in 3–5 days.

Rare: *Seizures, paralytic ileus, orthostatic hypotension, QTc prolongation, hepatic failure, increased intraocular pressure, hyponatremia, induction of mania, and activation of suicidal ideation in those under 24.*

Monitoring: EKG if over 50 years old. Associated with weight gain, determine BMI and metabolic risk before starting.

Pearl: Usually given with food while titrating. Once at an established dose, it is given at night to avoid daytime sedation.

Contraindications: Taking MAO-I, thioridazine, pimozide, or tamoxifen. Recovering from myocardial infarction. History of QTc prolongation, recent MI, or uncompensated heart failure [4].

Fluoxetine (Prozac)

Starting Dose: 20 mg PO daily. 10 mg PO daily can be used in elderly.

Titration: Increase by 20 mg PO daily every week. Wait for 4–6 weeks for the response when initializing therapy.

Max Dose: 120 mg PO daily.

FDA Approval: MDD (8 and older), OCD (7 and older), PMDD, bulimia, panic disorder.

Common Side Effects: GI upset, sexual dysfunction, insomnia, agitation, headache, nausea better in 3–5 days.

Rare: *Seizures, hyponatremia, induction of mania, and activation of suicidal ideation in those under 24.*

Monitoring: ECG if QT prolongation. Height and weight on children.

Pearl: No need to taper due to long half-life.

Contraindications: Taking MAO-I, thioridazine, pimozide, or tamoxifen [5].

Fluvoxamine (Luvox)

Starting Dose: 50 mg PO nightly.

Titration: Increase by 50 mg PO nightly every week.

Max Dose: 450 mg PO daily.

FDA Approval: Obsessive compulsive disorder and social anxiety disorder.

Common Side Effects: GI upset, sexual dysfunction, sweating, insomnia, agitation, headache, nausea better in 3–5 days.

Rare: *Seizures, hyponatremia, induction of mania, and activation of suicidal ideation in those under 24.*

Monitoring: None.

Pearl: Usually given at night due to sedation. Doses greater than 100 mg can be twice daily dosing to improve tolerability.

Contraindications: Taking MAO-I, thioridazine, pimozide, or tamoxifen [6].

Paroxetine (Paxil)

Starting Dose:

Immediate Release: 20 mg PO daily. 10 mg PO daily can be used in elderly.

Controlled Release: 25 mg PO daily.

Titration:

Immediate Release: Increase by 10 mg PO daily, after 1 week. Wait for 4–6 weeks for the response when initializing therapy.

Controlled Release: 12.5 mg po daily, after 1 week. Wait for 4–6 weeks for the response when initializing therapy.

Max Dose:

Immediate Release: 100 mg PO daily.

Controlled Release: 62.5 mg po daily.

FDA Approval: MDD, OCD, panic disorder, SAD, PTSD, GAD, PMDD.

Common Side Effects: GI upset, sexual dysfunction, agitation, headache, sedation, dizziness, tremor, bruising, weight gain, nausea (better in 3–5 days).

Rare: *Seizures, hyponatremia, induction of mania, serotonin syndrome, bleeding, SIADH, and activation of suicidal ideation in those under 24.*

Pearl: It may need to wean over several months for those who cannot tolerate withdrawal effects.

Contraindications: Taking MAO-I, thioridazine, pimozide, or tamoxifen.

Black Box Warning: Use may increase suicidal thoughts in children, adolescents, and young adults (24 and younger) [7, 8].

*****Beers List for drugs to avoid in the elderly*****

Sertraline (Zoloft)

Starting Dose: 50 mg PO daily. 25 mg PO daily in elderly.

Titration: Increase by 25–50 mg PO daily every week. Wait for 4–6 weeks for the response when initializing therapy.

Max Dose: 400 mg PO daily.

FDA Approval: Major depressive disorder (MDD), obsessive compulsive disorder (OCD), panic disorder, posttraumatic stress disorder (PTSD), premenstrual dysphoric disorder (PMDD), social anxiety disorder (SAD).

Common Side Effects: GI upset, sexual dysfunction, agitation, headache.

Rare: *Seizures, hyponatremia, induction of mania, hypotension, and activation of suicidal ideation in those under 24.*

Contraindications: Taking MAO-I, thioridazine, pimozide, or tamoxifen. Do not use Zoloft oral concentrate if the patient is taking disulfiram [9].

References

1. Caplan J, Stern T. Mnemonics in a mnutshell: 32 aids to psychiatric diagnosis. Curr Psychiatr Ther. 2008;7(10):27–33.
2. American Psychiatric Association. Anxiety disorders. In: Diagnostic and statistical manual of mental disorders (5th-TR). Washington, DC: American Psychiatric Association; 2022.
3. Jiao X, Qinjain H, Xingyu M, Minhan D, Yulu W, Yigou T, Min X, Qiang W. Optimal dose of serotonin reuptake inhibitors for obsessive-compulsive disorder in adults: a systematic review and dose–response

meta-analysis. National Library of Medicine. 2023, September 23. Retrieved April 12, 2024, from https://www.ncbi.nlm.nih.gov/pmc/articles/PMC8495022/.
4. Mallinckrodt LLC. Anafranil: highlights of prescribing information; 2012. https://www.accessdata.fda.gov/drugsatfda_docs/label/2012/019906s037lbl.pdf.
5. Eli Lilly and Company. Prozac: highlights of prescribing information; 1987. https://pi.lilly.com/us/prozac.pdf.
6. Jazz Pharmaceuticals. Luvox: highlights of prescribing information; 2007. https://www.accessdata.fda.gov/drugsatfda_docs/label/2008/022235lbl.pdf.
7. GlaxoSmithKline. Paxil: prescribing information; 2008. https://www.accessdata.fda.gov/drugsatfda_docs/label/2008/020031s060,020936s037,020710s024lbl.pdf.
8. GlaxoSmithKline. Paxil CR: prescribing information; 2014. https://www.accessdata.fda.gov/drugsatfda_docs/label/2014/020936s049lbl.pdf.
9. Pfizer. Zoloft: highlights of prescribing information; 2021. https://labeling.pfizer.com/ShowLabeling.aspx?id=517.

Insomnia

6

Contents

Insomnia

Insomnia is a common sleep disorder that millions of Americans experience each year. It is hallmarked by difficulty falling asleep, difficulty maintaining sleep, or early morning awakenings with the inability to go back to sleep. Insomnia may be short term lasting a few days to a week or a chronic condition lasting more than a month to years. It typically affects daytime activity leaving the person fatigued.

B. Floyd, T. Kane, *The Clinician's Guide to Common Psychiatric Disorders*, https://doi.org/10.1007/978-3-031-67958-2_6

Diagnosing and Monitoring

DSM-5-TR

Insomnia is defined as a dissatisfaction with sleep quality or quantity. Typically there is an issue with one or more of the following: Difficulty falling asleep, difficulty continuing sleep uninterrupted, and/or waking up early in the morning and not being able to go back to sleep. The sleep disturbances have to affect the patient at least three nights a week for at least 3 months. The sleep disturbances have to affect the quality of life of the patient. Finally, the insomnia cannot be explained by another sleep-wake disorder, physiological effect of a drug, and not better explained by another mental illness [1, p. 409].

Differential Diagnosis: Mood disorder, anxiety disorder, substance-related disorder, ADHD, OCD, alcohol use, cardiac illness, parasomnias, GI disorders, obstructive pulmonary disease, medication side effects, sleep apnea, RLS, chronic pain, stress reaction, active substance use (caffeine and stimulants).

Risk Factors: Older age, female gender, history of insomnia, significant stress, shift work, genetic, high pattern use of substances (caffeine/stimulants, alcohol, benzodiazepines).

Labs to Consider: CBC, chemistry profile, thyroid function, ferritin level if RLS, B12, and drugs of abuse if suspected.

Screening Scales

Pittsburgh Sleep Quality Index (PSQI): It is a self-reported questionnaire that takes between 5 and 10 min to complete. It consists of 19 questions covering seven components of sleep that produces a global score. The questionnaire also has five additional questions for bed partner that does not total into the final score.

Sleep Quality Scale: It is a self-reported questionnaire consisting of 28 questions evaluating 6 domains of sleep quality including daytime symptoms, restoration after sleep, problems initiating and maintaining sleep, difficulty waking, and sleep satisfaction. It is validated for ages 18–59.

Insomnia Severity Index: Self-reported questionnaire that consists of seven questions using a 0–4 severity rating. It helps determine severity of insomnia, impact on daily activity, and response to treatment.

STOP BANG: It is a self-report questionnaire consisting of eight questions that help determine risk of obstructive sleep apnea (OSA). It should be included when assessing for insomnia in individuals with known risk factors.

Treatment

First-line treatment of insomnia is sleep hygiene. Developing a nightly routine that involves consistent bedtimes and nightly rituals will prepare the mind for a restful night's sleep. Non-pharmacological therapy also involves CBT. When deciding on pharmacological therapy, it is important to consider the type of insomnia and duration of treatment and assess prior history of substance dependency before prescribing medications with abuse potential.

Sleep Hygiene

Sleep hygiene is the first step in treating insomnia. It should be implemented before all other interventions. Good sleep hygiene includes the following:

- Avoiding alcohol and caffeine before bed.
- Avoiding daytime napping
- Avoiding bright light (blue light) before bed
- Creating a consistent bedtime routine
- Using the bed only for sleep and sex

Cognitive Behavioral Therapy

First-line treatment involves cognitive behavioral therapy for primary insomnia in adults. It can be used in conjunction with sleep medication for maximum efficacy. Even those already on a medication for sleep can benefit from CBT. The types of CBT are stimulus control therapy and sleep restriction therapy.

Medications Based on Type of Insomnia

Sleep onset insomnia	Eszopiclone, ramelteon, zolpidem, zaleplon, zolpidem
Sleep maintenance Insomnia	Doxepin eszopiclone, suvorexant, zolpidem CR
Avoid in insomnia	Diphenhydramine, melatonin, mirtazapine, tiagabine, trazodone, tryptophan, and valerian.

Non-hypnotic Medications

Doxepin (Silenor)

Starting Dose: 3 mg PO nightly.

Titration: Increase by 3 mg PO nightly.

Max Dose: 6 mg typical for insomnia. Max dose is 300 mg/day.

FDA Approval: Sleep maintenance insomnia, depression, and anxiety associated with alcoholism and organic disease, psychotic depressive disorders with associated anxiety, involutional depression, manic-depressive disorder, and psychoneurotic patients with depression and/or anxiety.

Common Side Effects: Sedation, increased appetite, nausea, diarrhea, heartburn, fatigue, weakness, headache, anxiety, sexual dysfunction, weight gain.

Uncommon: *Paralytic ileus, hyperthermia, lowered seizure threshold, orthostatic hypotension, Arrythmias, QTc prolongation, hepatic failure, rare induction of mania.*

Monitoring: EKG prior to administering if over 50, taking QTc prolonging drugs, or certain cardiac conditions. Weight before initiating and following BMI every 3 months.

Contraindications: History of QTc prolongation, recent myocardial infarction, uncompensated heart failure, angle-closure glaucoma, severe urinary retention, taking drugs that inhibit TCA metabolism.

Black Box Warning: Use may increase suicidal thoughts in children, adolescents, and young adults (24 and younger) [2].

*****Beers List for drugs to avoid (>6 mg) in the elderly*****

Ramelteon (Rozerem): Melatonin 1 and 2 Receptor Agonist

Starting Dose: 8 mg PO nightly.

Titration: None.

Max Dose: 8 mg.

FDA Approval: Sleep onset insomnia.

Common Side Effects: Sedation, dizziness, fatigue, headache, respiratory depression, angioedema.

Rare: *Angioedema, respiratory depression when taken with other CNS depressants in overdose.*

Monitoring: None.

Contraindications: Hepatic impairment.

PEARL: Use may be titrated up by 8 mg prior to calling medication trial a failure. The only approved dose is 8 mg per night [3].

Non-benzodiazepine Hypnotics

Daridorexant (QUVIVIQ): Dual Orexin Receptor Antagonist/Hypnotic

Starting Dose: 25 mg PO nightly.

Titration: 25 mg PO nightly after 7 days.

Max Dose: 50 mg per night.

FDA Approval: Insomnia (sleep maintenance and sleep onset).

Common Side Effects: Sedation, headache.

Uncommon/Rare: Sleep paralysis, hypnagogic/hypnopompic hallucinations, symptoms similar to mild cataplexy.

Monitoring: None.

Contraindications: Narcolepsy, not recommended for someone taking a strong CYP450 3A4 inhibitor.

PEARL: It is not restricted to short-term use. Do not use it unless there is 7 h before needing to wake. The maximum dose is 25 mg in those taking mild CYP450 3A4 inhibitors [4].

Eszopiclone (Lunesta)

Starting Dose: 1 mg PO nightly.

Titration: 1 mg PO nightly every week.

Max Dose: 3 mg PO nightly.

FDA Approval: Insomnia.

Common Side Effects: Unpleasant taste, sedation, headache, dizziness, dry mouth, dose-dependent amnesia,

Uncommon: *Respiratory depression, angioedema.*

Monitoring: None.

Contraindications: Patient has experienced episodes of complex sleep behaviors while taking sleep medication [5].

Beers List for drugs to avoid >90 days in the elderly

Lemborexant (Dayvigo): Dual Orexin Receptor Antagonist/Hypnotic

Starting Dose: 5 mg PO nightly.

Titration: 5 mg PO nightly after 7 days.

Max Dose: 10 mg per night.

FDA Approval: Insomnia (sleep maintenance and sleep onset).

Common Side Effects: Sedation, headache, dizziness, abnormal dreams, sleep paralysis, hypnagogic/hypnopompic hallucinations.

Rare: Sleep paralysis, hypnagogic/hypnopompic hallucinations, symptoms similar to mild cataplexy.

Monitoring: None.

Contraindications: Narcolepsy, not recommended in someone taking a strong CYP450 3A4 inhibitor.

PEARL: It is not restricted to short-term use. Do not use it unless there is 7 h before needing to wake. The maximum dose is 5 mg in those taking mild CYP450 3A4 inhibitors [6].

Suvorexant (Belsomra): Dual Orexin Receptor Antagonist/Hypnotic

Starting Dose: 10 mg PO nightly.

Titration: 5 mg PO nightly after 7 days.

Max Dose: 20 mg per night.

FDA Approval: Insomnia (sleep maintenance and sleep onset).

Common Side Effects: Sedation, headache, abnormal dreams.

Rare: Sleep paralysis, hypnagogic/hypnopompic hallucinations, symptoms similar to mild cataplexy.

Monitoring: None.

Contraindications: Narcolepsy, not recommended in someone taking a strong or moderate CYP450 3A4 inhibitor.

PEARL: It is not restricted to short-term use. Do not use it unless there is 7 h before needing to wake [7].

Zaleplon (Sonata)

Starting Dose: 10 mg PO nightly.

Titration: Use may be increased to 20 mg PO nightly.

Max Dose: 20 mg PO nightly.

FDA Approval: Short-term treatment of insomnia.

Common Side Effects: Sedation, headache, dizziness, ataxia, dose-dependent amnesia, respiratory depression, angioedema.

Rare: *Respiratory depression when taken with other CNS depressants in overdose, angioedema.*

Monitoring: None.

Contraindications: Pt has experienced episode of complex sleep behaviors while taking a sleep.

PEARL: Patient with lower bodyweight may only require 5 mg nightly [8].

*****Beers List for drugs to avoid >90 days in the elderly*****

Zolpidem (Ambien)

Starting Dose: 10 mg PO nightly for men/5 mg PO nightly for women.

Titration: N/A.

Max Dose: 10 mg PO nightly.

FDA Approval: Short-term treatment of insomnia (7–10 days).

Common Side Effects: Sedation, headache, dizziness, dry mouth, dose-dependent amnesia.

Rare: *Respiratory depression* especially when taken with other CNS depressants in overdose, *angioedema*, and hallucinations.

Monitoring: None.

Contraindications: Pt has experienced episodes of complex sleep behaviors while taking a sleep medication [9].

*****Beers List for drugs to avoid >90 days in the elderly*****

Zolpidem (Ambien CR)

Starting Dose: 12.5 mg PO nightly for men/6.25 mg PO nightly for women.

Titration: N/A.

Max Dose: 12.5 mg PO nightly.

FDA Approval: Short-term treatment of insomnia (7–10 days).

Common Side Effects: Sedation, headache, dizziness, dry mouth, dose-dependent amnesia.

Rare: *Respiratory depression* especially when taken with other CNS depressants in overdose, *angioedema*, and hallucinations.

Monitoring: None.

Contraindications: Pt has experienced episodes of complex sleep behaviors while taking a sleep medication [10].

*****Beers List for drugs to avoid >90 days in the elderly*****

Zolpidem (Intermezzo)

Starting Dose: 3.5 mg sublingual nightly in men, 1.75 mg sublingual nightly in women and elderly.

Titration: N/A.

Max Dose: 10 mg sublingual nightly.

FDA Approval: Short-term treatment of insomnia (7–10 days).

Common Side Effects: Sedation, headache, dizziness, dry mouth, dose-dependent amnesia.

Rare: *Respiratory depression* especially when taken with other CNS depressants in overdose, *angioedema*, and hallucinations.

Monitoring: None.

Contraindications: Pt has experienced episodes of complex sleep behaviors while taking a sleep medication.

PEARL: Taken in the middle of the night if 4 h of bedtime remain [11].

*****Beers List for drugs to avoid >90 days in the elderly*****

Benzodiazepine Hypnotics

Temazepam (Restoril)

Starting Dose: 15 mg PO nightly.

Titration: 15 mg if tolerated but ineffective.

Max Dose: 30 mg PO nightly.

FDA Approval: Short-term treatment of insomnia (7–10 days).

Common Side Effects: Sedation, fatigue, depression, dizziness, ataxia, slurred speech, weakness, forgetfulness, confusion, hyperexcitability, nervousness, hypersalivation, dry mouth, rebound insomnia.

Rare: *Respiratory depression*, hallucinations, mania, *hypotension*, *hepatic dysfunction*, *renal dysfunction*, and blood dyscrasias.

Monitoring: None.

Contraindications: Pregnancy, angle-closure glaucoma, allergy.

PEARL: It is usually not written for more than a 1 month supply. DO NOT MIX with alcohol or opioids [12].

*****Beers List for drugs to avoid in the elderly*****

Dual-Purpose Adjuncts

Mirtazapine (Remeron)

Starting Dose: 7.5 mg PO nightly.

Titration: Increase to 15 mg PO nightly and then increase by 15 mg per titration.

Max Dose: Typically, 45 mg PO nightly.

FDA Approval: MDD.

Common Side Effects: Dry mouth, sedation, abnormal dreams, hypotension, change in urinary function, and flu-like symptoms.

Rare: *Seizures, induction of mania.*

Monitoring: PHQ-9.

PEARL: More sedating at lower doses with 7.5 mg being most sedating. It is often used for insomnia. Weight gain can be significant.

Black Box Warning: Use may increase suicidal thoughts in children, adolescents, and young adults (24 and younger) [13].

*****Beers List to be used with caution in the elderly*****

Trazodone (Desyrel)

Starting Dose: Insomnia: 25–50 mg. Depression: 150 mg in divided doses.

Titration: Insomnia: Increase by 50 mg PO nightly. Depression: Increase by 50 mg PO nightly.

Max Dose: 400 mg PO daily. Insomnia dose typically 50–150 mg PO nightly.

FDA Approval: MDD.

Common Side Effects: GI upset, blurred vision, constipation, dry mouth, dizziness, sedation, fatigue, headaches, sinus bradycardia with long-term use, hypotension, syncope, incoordination, tremor, nausea better in 3–5 days.

Rare: Rash, *priapism, seizures, induction of mania.*

Monitoring: PHQ-9.

PEARL: Often used for insomnia due to sedating properties at lower doses.

Black Box Warning: Use may increase suicidal thoughts in children, adolescents, and young adults (24 and younger) [14].

References

1. American Psychiatric Association. Sleep-Wake disorders. In: Diagnostic and statistical manual of mental disorders (5th-TR). Washington, DC: American Psychiatric Association; 2022.
2. Currax™ Pharmaceuticals LLC. Silenor: highlights of prescribing information; 2020. https://www.accessdata.fda.gov/drugsatfda_docs/label/2020/022036s006lbl.pdf.
3. Takeda Pharmaceuticals America, Inc. Rozarem: highlights of prescribing information; 2018. https://www.accessdata.fda.gov/drugsatfda_docs/label/2018/021782s021lbl.pdf.
4. Idorsia Pharmaceuticals US Inc. QUVIVIQ: highlights of prescribing information; 2022. https://www.idorsia.us/dam/jcr:57357654-064f-4333-ab0b-6b0bed5a79e4/Quviviq_PI.pdf.
5. Sunovion Pharmaceuticals Inc. Lunesta: highlights of prescribing information; 2014. https://www.accessdata.fda.gov/drugsatfda_docs/label/2014/021476s030lbl.pdf.
6. Eisai R&D Management Co., Ltd. Dayvigo: highlights of prescribing information; 2023. https://www.dayvigo.com/-/media/Files/DAYVIGO/PDF/prescribing-information.pdf?hash=b773622b-b11d-419e-9dee-068c55a90aab.
7. Merck Sharp & Dohme Corp. Belsomra: highlights of prescribing information; 2014. https://www.accessdata.fda.gov/drugsatfda_docs/label/2014/204569s000lbledt.pdf.

8. Pfizer, Inc. Sonata prescriber's information; 2023. https://labeling.pfizer.com/ShowLabeling.aspx?id=710.
9. Sanofi-Aventis U.S. LLC. Ambien: highlights of prescribing information; 2008. https://www.accessdata.fda.gov/drugsatfda_docs/label/2008/019908s027lbl.pdf.
10. Sanofi-Aventis U.S. LLC. Ambien CR: highlights of prescribing information; 2019. https://www.accessdata.fda.gov/drugsatfda_docs/label/2019/021774s027lbl.pdf.
11. Purdue Pharma L.P. Intermezzo: highlights of prescribing information; 2012. https://www.accessdata.fda.gov/drugsatfda_docs/label/2013/022328s001lbl.pdf.
12. Mallinckrodt Inc. Restoril prescribing information; 2017. https://www.drugs.com/pro/restoril.html.
13. Merck & Co., Inc. Remeron: highlights of prescribing information; 2021. https://www.accessdata.fda.gov/drugsatfda_docs/label/2021/020415s038,021208s028lbl.pdf.
14. Pragma Pharmaceuticals, LLC. Deseryl: highlights of prescribing information; 2017. https://www.accessdata.fda.gov/drugsatfda_docs/label/2017/018207s032lbl.pdf.

Posttraumatic Stress Disorder (PTSD) 7

Contents

B. Floyd, T. Kane, *The Clinician's Guide to Common Psychiatric Disorders*, https://doi.org/10.1007/978-3-031-67958-2_7

Posttraumatic Stress Disorder (PTSD)

Posttraumatic Stress Disorder (PTSD) is a psychiatric disorder that may develop after an individual is exposed to a traumatic/terrifying event. It can be directly experiencing it, witnessing it, or learning about the event that happened to a close friend or family member. It is hallmarked by intrusive thoughts about the event, avoidance of triggering situations that remind the person of the event, irritability/anger, and changes in mood and cognition.

Diagnosing and Monitoring

*Mnemonic: **Trauma:*** **T**raumatic event, **R**eexperiencing trauma, **A**voiding traumatic memories, **U**nable to function (negative cognition), **M**onth or more of symptoms, **A**rousal increased.

DSM-5-TR

Posttraumatic Stress Disorder in Individuals Older Than 6 Years

The DSM-5-TR lists PTSD as a result of exposure to actual or threatened death, serious injury, or sexual violence by experiencing it directly, witnessing it occurs to others, or learning that it happened to a close family member or friend. The following criteria must also be met [1, p. 301]:

1 or more Intrusive Symptom: Intrusive memories, nightmares, dissociative reaction, psychological distress at exposure, and physiological reaction to cues that symbolize aspect of trauma.

1 or more Avoidance Symptom: Efforts to avoid distressing memories, thoughts, or feelings of event and efforts to avoid external reminders that arouse memories, thoughts, or feelings about event.

2 or more Negative Symptoms: Inability to remember aspects of trauma, negative beliefs, blaming others or self, persistent negative emotional state, markedly diminished interest or participation

in significant activities, feelings of detachment or estrangement, and inability to experience positive emotions.

2 or more Arousal Symptoms: Irritable or angry outbursts, self-destructive behavior, hypervigilance, exaggerated startle response, problems with concentration, or sleep disturbances.

Symptoms have occurred for at least 1 month. It is not caused by the physiological effects of a substance and cannot be better explained by another mental illness.

Differential Diagnosis: Adjustment disorder, brief psychotic disorder, acute stress disorder, and intrusive thoughts associated with OCD.

Risk Factors: Experienced or witnessed trauma, strong genetic etiology component and tends to run in families, MDD in first-degree relative. Other pre- and peri-trauma risk factors include gender, race, age, socioeconomic status, prior support system, and childhood adversity.

Labs to Consider: Nonspecific.

Screening Scales

***PTSD Checklist for DSM-5 (PCL-5)*: It is a** three-part questionnaire that covers most prevalent traumatic events. Part 3 is graded and is a 20-question self-report where the patient rates 20 common PTSD symptoms from 0 (Not at all) to 4 (Extremely). It can be used to continue to monitor symptoms throughout treatment. Cutoff score of 31–33 is suggestive of PTSD.

Impact of Events Scale Revised (IES-R): It is a self-reported questionnaire consisting of 22 questions covering common PTSD symptoms. Severity is rated 0 (Not at all) to 4 (Extremely). Total score is calculated and a cut-off score of 33 is indicative of probable PTSD.

Short Posttraumatic Stress Disorder Rating Interview (SPRINT): It is an 8-item self-reported scale covering core symptoms of PTSD. Severity is rated from 0 (Not at all) to 4 (Very much). Cut-off score of 14 warrants further investigation into PTSD diagnosis.

Treatment

PTSD is a complex disorder with a wide array of symptoms. It is hallmarked by high levels of anxiety that can manifest as irritability, anger, and insomnia. There is not one treatment modality for PTSD and not one class of medication that will work on all symptoms. Trauma-informed CBT and Eye Movement Desensitization and Reprocessing (EMDR) have shown success in treating PTSD. Therapy coupled with medication management shows superior efficacy than either treatment alone.

Non-pharmacologic Interventions

Trauma-Focused CBT (TF-CBT): Geared towards children, adolescents, and families, TF-CBT's goal is to create a life worth living after trauma occurs. It is a short-term treatment lasting roughly 12 sessions. It combines trauma-sensitive interventions with principles of cognitive behavioral therapy.

Trauma-Informed CBT: Classical CBT in which the therapist assumes their patient could have a trauma history and will take steps to avoid triggering the individual. Not all CBT therapists are trauma informed.

Eye Movement Desensitization and Reprocessing (EMDR): Classically, the patient would detail their traumatic history with the therapist while following a light running horizontally with their eyes. It has evolved into hand paddles that will vibrate in alternating hands or the patient may use "tappers" while they recount the event. Repeated exposure to the event while engaging both sides of the brain begins to desensitize the patient from their memories so they become less triggering.

Pharmacologic Interventions

First-Line Medications

Paroxetine (Paxil)

Starting Dose: Immediate Release: 20 mg PO daily. Controlled Release: 25 mg PO daily. 10 mg PO daily can be used in elderly.

Titration: Immediate Release: Increase by 10 mg PO daily every week. Controlled Release: 12.5 mg po daily. Wait for 4–6 weeks for the response when initializing therapy.

Max Dose: Immediate Release: 50 mg PO daily. Controlled Release: 62.5 mg po daily.

FDA Approval: MDD, OCD, panic disorder, SAD, PTSD, GAD, PMDD.

Common Side Effects: GI upset, sexual dysfunction, agitation, headache, nausea better in 3–5 days.

Rare: *Seizures, hyponatremia, induction of mania, and activation of suicidal ideation in those under 24.*

Monitoring: PHQ-9.

Pearl: There is a need to wean over several months for those who cannot tolerate withdrawal effects.

Contraindications: Taking MAO-I, thioridazine, pimozide, or tamoxifen.

Black Box Warning: Use may increase suicidal thoughts in children, adolescents, and young adults (24 and younger) [2].

*****Beers List for drugs to avoid in the elderly*****

Sertraline (Zoloft)

Starting Dose: 50 mg PO daily. 25 mg PO daily in elderly.

Titration: Increase by 25–50 mg PO daily every week. Wait for 4–6 weeks for the response when initializing therapy.

Max Dose: 200 mg PO daily.

FDA Approval: Major depressive disorder (MDD), obsessive compulsive disorder (OCD), panic disorder, posttraumatic stress disorder (PTSD), premenstrual dysphoric disorder (PMDD), social anxiety disorder (SAD).

Common Side Effects: GI upset, sexual dysfunction, agitation, headache.

Rare: *Seizures, hyponatremia, induction of mania, hypotension, and activation of suicidal ideation in those under 24.*

Monitoring: PHQ-9.

Contraindications: Taking MAO-I, thioridazine, pimozide, or tamoxifen.

Black Box Warning: Use may increase suicidal thoughts in children, adolescents, and young adults (24 and younger) [3].

****Other SSRI/SNRI that are used but not FDA approved include citalopram, desvenlafaxine, escitalopram, fluoxetine, fluvoxamine, and venlafaxine. ****

Off-Label Treatment for Hyperarousal/Nightmares

Clonidine (Catapres)

Starting Dose: 0.1 mg PO daily.

Titration: Increase by 0.1 mg PO daily every week.

Max Dose: 0.4 mg/day.

FDA Approval: Hypertension, ADHD in children 6–17 years old.

Common Side Effects: Sedation, dizziness, abdominal pain, nausea, fatigue, weakness, hypotension, dry mouth, constipation, and bradycardia.

Rare: *Sinus bradycardia, atrioventricular block. Hypertensive encephalopathy*, *CVA*, and *death* (during withdrawal).

Monitoring: Blood pressure regularly [4].

*****Beers List for drugs to avoid in the elderly*****

Prazosin (Minipress)

Starting Dose: 1 mg PO nightly.

Titration: Increase by 1–2 mg PO nightly every couple weeks.

Max Dose: 40 mg/day.

FDA Approval: Hypertension.

Common Side Effects: Dizziness, lightheadedness, headache, fatigue, blurred vision, nausea, orthostatic hypotension, *syncope with sudden loss of consciousness.*

Rare: *Priapism.*

Monitoring: None.

Pearl: Given at night to treat nightmares. It may also be given during the day to help combat hyperarousal [5].

Beers List for drugs to avoid in the elderly

Irritability Off-Label Adjuncts

Quetiapine (Seroquel)

Starting Dose: 50 mg PO BID.

Titration: 100 mg/day. Once at 400 mg/day, it may increase by 200 mg/day.

Max Dose: 800 mg PO daily.

FDA Approval: MDD, bipolar depression, bipolar maintenance, schizophrenia.

Common Side Effects: GI upset, sexual dysfunction, insomnia, agitation, sedation, dizziness, urinary retention, headache, weight loss, myalgia, sweating, anorexia, hypertension, and nausea better in 3–5 days.

Rare: *Neuroleptic malignant syndrome, seizures.*

Monitoring: PHQ-9, BMI every 3 months, lipid panel, and A1c annually. Waist circumference, blood pressure, fasting plasma glucose, and fasting lipid profile prior to start, within 3 months, and then annually. AIMS score every 3–6 months.

Pearl: Known for its sedating properties, it could be useful as an insomnia adjunct in doses up to 100 mg.

Black Box Warning: Elderly dementia patients who take Seroquel have a higher risk of death. Use may increase suicidal thoughts in children, adolescents, and young adults (24 and younger) [6].

Risperidone (Risperdal)

Starting Dose: 0.5 mg PO BID (1 mg/day).

Titration: Increase by 1 mg/day, every day.

Max Dose: 16 mg/day.

FDA Approval: Schizophrenia, acute mania/mixed mania, autism-related irritability in children, and bipolar maintenance.

Common Side Effects: Increased risk for diabetes and dyslipidemia, drug-induced parkinsonism, hyperprolactinemia, dizziness, insomnia, anxiety, sedation, GI distress, weight gain, sexual dysfunction, tardive dyskinesia, and orthostatic hypotension.

Uncommon/Rare: *Hyperglycemia, neuroleptic malignant syndrome, seizures.*

Monitoring: PHQ-9, BMI every 3 months, lipid panel, and A1c annually. Waist circumference, blood pressure, fasting plasma glucose, and fasting lipid profile prior to start, within 3 months, and then annually.

Black Box Warning: Elderly dementia patients who take Zyprexa have a higher risk of death. Use may increase suicidal thoughts in children, adolescents, and young adults (24 and younger) [7].

Insomnia

Non-hypnotic Medications

Doxepin (Silenor)

Starting Dose: 3 mg PO nightly.

Titration: Increase by 3 mg PO nightly.

Max Dose: 6 mg typical for insomnia. Max dose is 300 mg/day.

FDA Approval: Sleep maintenance insomnia, depression and anxiety associated with alcoholism and organic disease, psychotic depressive disorders with associated anxiety, involutional depression, manic-depressive disorder, and psychoneurotic patients with depression and/or anxiety.

Common Side Effects: Sedation, increased appetite, nausea, diarrhea, heartburn, fatigue, weakness, headache, anxiety, sexual dysfunction, weight gain.

Uncommon: *Paralytic ileus, hyperthermia, lowered seizure threshold, orthostatic hypotension, Arrythmias, QTc prolongation, hepatic failure, rare induction of mania.*

Monitoring: EKG prior to administering if over 50, taking QTc prolonging drugs, or certain cardiac conditions. Weight before initiating and following BMI every 3 months.

Contraindications: History of QTc prolongation, recent myocardial infarction, uncompensated heart failure, angle-closure glaucoma, severe urinary retention, taking drugs that inhibit TCA metabolism.

Black Box Warning: Use may increase suicidal thoughts in children, adolescents, and young adults (24 and younger) [8].

*****Beers List for drugs to avoid (>6 mg) in the elderly*****

Ramelteon (Rozerem): Melatonin 1 and 2 Receptor Agonist

Starting Dose: 8 mg PO nightly.

Titration: None.

Max Dose: 8 mg.

FDA Approval: Sleep onset insomnia.

Common Side Effects: Sedation, dizziness, fatigue, headache, respiratory depression, angioedema.

Rare: *Angioedema, respiratory depression when taken with other CNS depressants in overdose.*

Monitoring: None.

Contraindications: Hepatic impairment.

PEARL: Titrate up by 8 mg prior to calling medication trial a failure. The only approved dose 8 mg per night [9].

Non-benzodiazepine Hypnotics

Daridorexant (QUVIVIQ): Dual Orexin Receptor Antagonist/Hypnotic

Starting Dose: 25 mg PO nightly.

Titration: 25 mg PO nightly after 7 days.

Max Dose: 50 mg per night.

FDA Approval: Insomnia (sleep maintenance and sleep onset).

Common Side Effects: Sedation, headache.

Uncommon/Rare: Sleep paralysis, hypnagogic/hypnopompic hallucinations, symptoms similar to mild cataplexy.

Monitoring: None.

Contraindications: Narcolepsy, not recommended for someone taking a strong CYP450 3A4 inhibitor.

PEARL: It is not restricted to short-term use. Do not use it unless there is 7 h before needing to wake. The maximum dose is 25 mg in those taking mild CYP450 3A4 inhibitors [10].

Eszopiclone (Lunesta)

Starting Dose: 1 mg PO nightly.

Titration: 1 mg PO nightly every week.

Max Dose: 3 mg PO nightly.

FDA Approval: Insomnia.

Common Side Effects: Unpleasant taste, sedation, headache, dizziness, dry mouth, dose-dependent amnesia.

Uncommon: Respiratory depression, angioedema.

Monitoring: None.

Contraindications: Patient has experienced episodes of complex sleep behaviors while taking sleep medication [11].

*****Beers List for drugs to avoid >90 days in the elderly*****

Lemborexant (Dayvigo): Dual Orexin Receptor Antagonist/Hypnotic

Starting Dose: 5 mg PO nightly.

Titration: 5 mg PO nightly after 7 days.

Max Dose: 10 mg per night.

FDA Approval: Insomnia (sleep maintenance and sleep onset).

Common Side Effects: Sedation, headache, dizziness, abnormal dreams, sleep paralysis, hypnagogic/hypnopompic hallucinations.

Rare: Sleep paralysis, hypnagogic/hypnopompic hallucinations, symptoms similar to mild cataplexy.

Monitoring: None.

Contraindications: Narcolepsy, not recommended in someone taking a strong CYP450 3A4 inhibitor.

PEARL: It is not restricted to short-term use. Do not use it unless there is 7 h before needing to wake. The maximum dose is 5 mg in those taking mild CYP450 3A4 inhibitors [12].

Suvorexant (Belsomra): Dual Orexin Receptor Antagonist/Hypnotic

Starting Dose: 10 mg PO nightly.

Titration: 5 mg PO nightly after 7 days.

Max Dose: 20 mg per night.

FDA Approval: Insomnia (sleep maintenance and sleep onset).

Common Side Effects: Sedation, headache, abnormal dreams.

Rare: Sleep paralysis, hypnagogic/hypnopompic hallucinations, symptoms similar to mild cataplexy.

Monitoring: None.

Contraindications: Narcolepsy, not recommended in someone taking a strong or moderate CYP450 3A4 inhibitor.

PEARL: It is not restricted to short term use. Do not use it unless there is 7 h before needing to wake [13].

Zaleplon (Sonata)

Starting Dose: 10 mg PO nightly.

Titration: May increase to 20 mg PO nightly.

Max Dose: 20 mg PO nightly.

FDA Approval: Short-term treatment of insomnia.

Common Side Effects: Sedation, headache, dizziness, ataxia, dose-dependent amnesia, respiratory depression, angioedema.

Rare: *Respiratory depression when taken with other CNS depressants in overdose, angioedema.*

Monitoring: None.

Contraindications: Pt has experienced episode of complex sleep behaviors while taking a sleep.

PEARL: Patient with lower bodyweight may only require 5 mg nightly [14].

*****Beers List for drugs to avoid >90 days in the elderly*****

Zolpidem (Ambien)

Starting Dose: 10 mg PO nightly for men/5 mg PO nightly for women.

Titration: N/A.

Max Dose: 10 mg PO nightly.

FDA Approval: Short-term treatment of insomnia (7–10 days).

Common Side Effects: Sedation, headache, dizziness, dry mouth, dose-dependent amnesia.

Rare: *Respiratory depression* especially when taken with other CNS depressants in overdose, *angioedema*, and hallucinations.

Monitoring: None.

Contraindications: Pt has experienced episodes of complex sleep behaviors while taking a sleep medication [15].

*****Beers List for druSgs to avoid >90 days in the elderly*****

Zolpidem (Ambien CR)

Starting Dose: 12.5 mg PO nightly for men/6.25 mg PO nightly for women.

Titration: N/A.

Max Dose: 12.5 mg PO nightly.

FDA Approval: Short-term treatment of insomnia (7–10 days).

Common Side Effects: Sedation, headache, dizziness, dry mouth, dose-dependent amnesia.

Rare: *Respiratory depression* especially when taken with other CNS depressants in overdose, *angioedema*, and hallucinations.

Monitoring: None.

Contraindications: Pt has experienced episodes of complex sleep behaviors while taking a sleep medication [16].

*****Beers List for drugs to avoid >90 days in the elderly*****

Zolpidem (Intermezzo)

Starting Dose: 3.5 mg sublingual nightly in men, 1.75 mg sublingual nightly in women and elderly.

Titration: N/A.

Max Dose: 10 mg sublingual nightly.

FDA Approval: Short-term treatment of insomnia (7–10 days).

Common Side Effects: Sedation, headache, dizziness, dry mouth, dose-dependent amnesia.

Rare: *Respiratory depression* especially when taken with other CNS depressants in overdose, *angioedema*, and hallucinations.

Monitoring: None.

Contraindications: Pt has experienced episodes of complex sleep behaviors while taking a sleep medication.

PEARL: Taken in the middle of the night if 4 h of bedtime remain [17].

*****Beers List for drugs to avoid >90 days in the elderly*****

Benzodiazepine Hypnotics

Temazepam (Restoril)

Starting Dose: 15 mg PO nightly.

Titration: 15 mg if tolerated but ineffective.

Max Dose: 30 mg PO nightly.

FDA Approval: Short-term treatment of insomnia (7–10 days).

Common Side Effects: Sedation, fatigue, depression, dizziness, ataxia, slurred speech, weakness, forgetfulness, confusion, hyperexcitability, nervousness, hypersalivation, dry mouth, rebound insomnia.

Rare: Respiratory depression, hallucinations, mania, hypotension, hepatic dysfunction, renal dysfunction, and blood dyscrasias.

Monitoring: None.

Contraindications: Pregnancy, angle-closure glaucoma, allergy.

PEARL: It is usually not written for more than a 1 month supply. DO NOT MIX with alcohol or opioids (Mallinckrodt Inc. 2017).

*****Beers List for drugs to avoid in the elderly*****

Dual Purpose Adjuncts

Mirtazapine (Remeron)

Starting Dose: 7.5 mg PO nightly.

Titration: Increase to 15 mg PO nightly and then increase by 15 mg per titration.

Max Dose: Typically, 45 mg PO nightly.

FDA Approval: MDD.

Common Side Effects: Dry mouth, sedation, abnormal dreams, hypotension, change in urinary function, and flu-like symptoms.

Rare: *Seizures, induction of mania.*

Monitoring: PHQ-9.

PEARL: More sedating at lower doses with 7.5 mg being most sedating. Often used for insomnia. Weight gain can be significant.

Black Box Warning: Use may increase suicidal thoughts in children, adolescents, and young adults (24 and younger) [18].

****Beers List to be used with caution in the elderly*****

Trazodone (Desyrel)

Starting Dose: Insomnia: 25–50 mg. Depression: 150 mg in divided doses.

Titration: Insomnia: Increase by 50 mg PO nightly. Depression: Increase by 50 mg PO nightly.

Max Dose: 400 mg PO daily. Insomnia dose typically 50–150 mg PO nightly.

FDA Approval: MDD.

Common Side Effects: GI upset, blurred vision, constipation, dry mouth, dizziness, sedation, fatigue, headaches, sinus bradycardia with long-term use, hypotension, syncope, incoordination, tremor, nausea better in 3–5 days.

Rare: Rash, *priapism, seizures, induction of mania.*

Monitoring: PHQ-9.

PEARL: It is often used for insomnia due to sedating properties at lower doses.

Black Box Warning: Use may increase suicidal thoughts in children, adolescents, and young adults (24 and younger) [19].

References

1. American Psychiatric Association. Trauma- and stressor-related disorders. In: Diagnostic and statistical manual of mental disorders (5th-TR). Washington, DC: American Psychiatric Association; 2022.
2. GlaxoSmithKline. Paxil: prescribing information; 2008. https://www.accessdata.fda.gov/drugsatfda_docs/label/2008/020031s060,020936s037,020710s024lbl.pdf.
3. Pfizer. Zoloft: highlights of prescribing information; 2021. https://labeling.pfizer.com/ShowLabeling.aspx?id=517.
4. Catapres: Package Insert. Drugs.com; n.d. Retrieved January 20, 2024, from https://www.drugs.com/pro/catapres.html.
5. Prazosin - FDA prescribing information, side effects and uses. n.d. Drugs.com. https://www.drugs.com/pro/prazosin.html.
6. AstraZeneca Pharmaceuticals LP. Seroquel: highlights of prescribing information; 2009. https://www.accessdata.fda.gov/drugsatfda_docs/label/2009/020639s045s046lbl.pdf.
7. Janssen Pharmaceutical Companies. Risperdal: highlights of prescribing information; 2007. https://www.accessdata.fda.gov/drugsatfda_docs/label/2019/020272s082,020588s070,021444s056lbl.pdf.
8. Currax™ Pharmaceuticals LLC. Silenor: highlights of prescribing information; 2020. https://www.accessdata.fda.gov/drugsatfda_docs/label/2020/022036s006lbl.pdf.
9. Takeda Pharmaceuticals America, Inc. Rozarem: highlights of prescribing information; 2018. https://www.accessdata.fda.gov/drugsatfda_docs/label/2018/021782s021lbl.pdf.
10. Idorsia Pharmaceuticals US Inc. QUVIVIQ: highlights of prescribing information; 2022. https://www.idorsia.us/dam/jcr:57357654-064f-4333-ab0b-6b0bed5a79e4/Quviviq_PI.pdf.
11. Sunovion Pharmaceuticals Inc. Lunesta: highlights of prescribing information; 2014. https://www.accessdata.fda.gov/drugsatfda_docs/label/2014/021476s030lbl.pdf.
12. Eisai R&D Management Co., Ltd. Dayvigo: highlights of prescribing information; 2023. https://www.dayvigo.com/-/media/Files/DAYVIGO/PDF/prescribing-information.pdf?hash=b773622b-b11d-419e-9dee-068c55a90aab.
13. Merck Sharp & Dohme Corp. Belsomra: highlights of prescribing information; 2014. https://www.accessdata.fda.gov/drugsatfda_docs/label/2014/204569s000lbledt.pdf.
14. Pfizer, Inc. Sonata prescriber's information; 2023. https://labeling.pfizer.com/ShowLabeling.aspx?id=710.
15. Sanofi-Aventis U.S. LLC. Ambien: highlights of prescribing information; 2008. https://www.accessdata.fda.gov/drugsatfda_docs/label/2008/019908s027lbl.pdf.

16. Sanofi-Aventis U.S. LLC. Ambien CR: highlights of prescribing information; 2019. https://www.accessdata.fda.gov/drugsatfda_docs/label/2019/021774s027lbl.pdf.
17. Purdue Pharma L.P. Intermezzo: highlights of prescribing information; 2012. https://www.accessdata.fda.gov/drugsatfda_docs/label/2013/022328s001lbl.pdf.
18. Merck & Co., Inc. Remeron: highlights of prescribing information; 2021. https://www.accessdata.fda.gov/drugsatfda_docs/label/2021/020415s038,021208s028lbl.pdf.
19. Pragma Pharmaceuticals, LLC. Deseryl: highlights of prescribing information; 2017. https://www.accessdata.fda.gov/drugsatfda_docs/label/2017/018207s032lbl.pdf.

Substance Use and Abuse 8

Contents

Alcohol Use Disorder

Alcohol use disorder is a chronic condition in which the patient has an uncontrollable dependence on alcohol despite it negatively affecting their life in various settings. During this period, the patient will experience alcohol intoxication and may experience withdrawal symptoms if they stop drinking abruptly. It is diagnosed in degrees of severity based on symptoms present.

B. Floyd, T. Kane, *The Clinician's Guide to Common Psychiatric Disorders*, https://doi.org/10.1007/978-3-031-67958-2_8

Diagnosing and Monitoring

CAGE Questionnaire: Generally, 2 or 3 “yes” answers suggest heavy alcohol use or alcohol use disorder. It can be adapted for other substance use.

- Have you ever felt you should ***C***ut down on your drinking (or drug use)?

- Have people ***A***nnoyed you by criticizing your drinking (or drug use)?
- Have you ever felt bad or ***G***uilty about your drinking (or drug use)?
- Have you ever had a drink (or used drugs) first thing in the morning to steady your nerves or get rid of a hangover (***E***ye-opener)?

It is no longer recommended by the USPSTF because it may miss prevention opportunities. It may consider the AUDIT tool or the Single Alcohol Screening Question (SASQ) [1].

DSM-5-TR

The DSM-5-TR lists alcohol use disorder as a problematic use of alcohol leading to significant decline of the quality of life with at least two of the following over the past year [2, p. 553]:

1. Consuming more alcohol than was intended.
2. Inability to cut back or quit using alcohol.
3. Excessive time used obtaining alcohol or recovering from its effects.
4. Cravings.
5. Failing to fulfill major role obligations at work, school, or home.
6. Continued use despite detrimental effects to social or interpersonal relationships.
7. Important social, occupational, or recreational activities are given up or reduced because of alcohol use.
8. Using alcohol when it is physically dangerous.

9. Alcohol use is continued despite knowledge of having a persistent or recurrent physical or psychological problem that is likely to have been caused or exacerbated by alcohol.
10. Tolerance.
11. Withdrawal.

Differential Diagnosis: MDD, bipolar, anxiety disorders, personality disorders, dysthymic disorder, insomnia, electrolyte imbalances, ketoacidosis, anti-social personality disorder, and conduct disorder in adolescents.

Risk Factors: Genetic loading (family history of substance abuse) associated with people who are heavy users, co-occurring psychiatric disorders, younger males, Native American and white ethnicity, other substance use disorders, chronic pain, and untreated pathological anxiety.

Labs to Consider: CBC, chemistry profile, thyroid function, B12. Possibly drug toxicity screening, BAC, liver function testing.

Screening Scales

Tobacco, Alcohol, Prescription Medication, and Other Substance Use (TAPS)—It provides screening and brief assessment of commonly used drugs. It can be self-administered or administered by a clinician. Part One asks screens for use in the previous 12 months. If there is a positive answer, then part two screens for use in the past 3 months. If two or more answers are "yes" in part Two, it is considered a positive screen with a 70% sensitivity for tobacco, alcohol, and marijuana.

The Alcohol, Smoking, and Substance Involvement Screening Test (ASSIST)—It is a clinician-driven screening assessment that screens for nine commonly abused substances. The first question screens for the drug and subsequent follow-up questions ask about frequency and attempts to cutback. Score is totaled, and based on the total, there is a chart for recommendations. This can be found on the World Health Organization's website.

The NIAAA Single Alcohol Screening Question (SASQ)—How many times in the past year have you had (4 for women, or 5 for men) or more drinks in a day? If the patient answers one or more, further screening should be completed.

Alcohol Use Disorders Identification Test Consumption (AUDIT-C)—It is an abbreviated version of the AUDIT tool. It focuses on consumption of alcohol and how often. It has three questions rated on a scale of 0–4 for a total possible score of 12. A score above 4 for men and 3 for women is positive. The higher the score, the higher the likelihood that there is problematic drinking.

Alcohol Symptom Checklist—It is an 11-question, self-reported screening tool that the patient fills out. The questions are based on DSM-5 criteria for AUD. It can help determine severity of AUD as well.

Treatment

Severity of alcohol use disorder determines the treatment. Those with mild AUD would likely benefit from psychosocial interventions such as alcohol counseling and mutual help groups. Those with moderate to severe AUD would most benefit from a combined approach with medication and psychosocial intervention. Those with limited insight may benefit from groups such as alcoholics anonymous. Psychosocial interventions include substance abuse education classes, substance abuse counseling program, alcoholics anonymous, family treatment, and possible admission to hospital or treatment center.

Non-pharmacologic Interventions

Cognitive Behavioral Therapy (CBT): It is a type of therapy that focuses on changing one's thoughts and behaviors to improve mood and functioning. It is a short-term, collaborative, goal-oriented therapy where the therapist helps the client identify negative thought patterns and behaviors, and they develop ways to reconceptualize these thoughts and behaviors into something more positive.

Combined Behavioral Intervention (CBI): The patient and behavior therapist work together to identify the problem, define the specifics of the problem, develop a plan for solving the problem, and evaluate different strategies for implementing the plan.

Alcoholics Anonymous (AA): There is a 12-step program set on spiritual principles. It is a fellowship of people trying to achieve and sustain sobriety. No cost to the patient and everyone is welcome.

Pharmacologic Interventions

Acamprosate (Campral)

Starting Dose: 666 mg PO three times a day.
Titration: Not required.
Max Dose: 666 mg PO three times a day.
FDA Approval: Maintenance of alcohol abstinence.
Common Side Effects: Diarrhea, nausea, anxiety, depression, suicidality.
Monitoring: None.
Contraindication: Renal impairment.
Pearl: It is best used for alcohol abstinence not goal of reduced drinking.
Black Box Warning: Liver damage or hepatitis (hepatotoxicity) [3].

Disulfiram (Antabuse)

Starting Dose: 250 mg PO daily.
Titration: 125–250 mg PO daily.
Max Dose: 500 mg PO daily.
FDA Approval: Maintenance of alcohol abstinence.
Common Side Effects: Flushing, headache, tachycardia, nausea, vomiting if consuming alcohol, metallic taste dermatitis, sedation,
Uncommon: *Myocardial infarction*, *congestive heart failure*, *respiratory depression*, *hepatotoxicity* if alcohol is consumed.
Monitoring: Baseline liver function test and then periodic testing afterwards.

Contraindications: If a patient is intoxicated, drank within the last 12 h, and has psychosis and cardiovascular disease, the patient may rely on certain medications: metronidazole, amprenavir, ritonavir, or sertraline.

Pearl: Do not take disulfiram until at least 12 h after drinking.

Black Box Warning: Never administer if a patient has alcohol intoxication or without the patient's full consent [4].

Naltrexone (Revia/Vivitrol)

Starting Dose: 50 mg PO daily. 380 mg every 4 weeks for injection (Vivitrol).

Titration: None.

Max Dose: 50 mg PO daily. 380 mg every 4 weeks for injection.

FDA Approval: Alcohol dependence, blockade effects of exogenously administered opioids, relapse prevention of opioid dependence.

Common Side Effects: Nausea, vomiting, decreased appetite, dizziness, injection site reactions, dysphoria, and anxiety.

Uncommon: *Eosinophilic pneumonia, hepatocellular injury at high doses, severe injection site reactions requiring surgery.*

Monitoring: Liver function prior to initiating treatment. Urine drug screen in certain cases to make sure no opioids in system.

Contraindication: Patients receiving opioid analgesics and current physiologic opioid dependence. In acute opioid withdrawal, patients who have failed the naloxone challenge test or have a positive urine screen for opioids, hypersensitivity to naltrexone, polylactide-co-glycolide (PLG), carboxymethylcellulose, or any other components of the diluent.

Pearl: Patients should have a medical alert bracelet for naltrexone use.

Black Box Warning: Liver damage or hepatitis (hepatotoxicity) [5, 6].

Off-Label

Topiramate (Topamax)

Starting Dose: 25 mg PO nightly.

Titration: Increase by 25 mg PO nightly every 7 days.
Max Dose:
FDA Approval: Seizures, Migraine prophylaxis, Chronic weight management.
Common Side Effects: Sedation, asthenia, dizziness, ataxia, paresthesia, nystagmus, nervousness, tremor, nausea, appetite loss, weight loss, blurred/double vision, confusion, memory problems, mood problems, fatigue, and taste disturbances.
Uncommon: *Metabolic ketoacidosis,* kidney stones, *hyperammonemia, rare SJS or purpura, hyperthermia, rare activation of suicidality.*
Monitoring: Baseline serum bicarbonate and then periodically, checking for hyperchloremic, non-anion gap metabolic acidosis.
Contraindications: Within a 6 h window of alcohol use, patients with metabolic acidosis while on metformin.
Pearl: Use has been shown to reduce the number of episodes of binge-drinking [7].

Tobacco Use Disorder

Tobacco use disorder is a chronic disorder where a person becomes dependent on nicotine, commonly found in cigarettes. The user will continue despite negative health consequences and social impact it may have on them. It is important to also rate the severity of the problem as this could help guide treatment.

Diagnosing and Monitoring

DSM-5-TR

The DSM-5-TR lists Alcohol Use Disorder as a problematic use of alcohol leading to significant decline of the quality of life with at least two of the following over the past year [2, p. 645]:

1. Consuming more tobacco than was intended.
2. Inability to cut back or quit using tobacco.

3. Excessive time used in obtaining tobacco or recovering from its effects.
4. Cravings.
5. Failing to fulfill major role obligations at work, school, or home.
6. Continued use despite detrimental effects to social or interpersonal relationships.
7. Important social, occupational, or recreational activities are given up or reduced because of tobacco use.
8. Using tobacco when it is physically dangerous.
9. Tobacco use is continued despite knowledge of having a persistent or recurrent physical or psychological problem that is likely to have been caused or exacerbated by tobacco.
10. Tolerance.
11. Withdrawal.

Differential Diagnoses: Depressive and anxiety disorders. Consider COPD, emphysema, angina pectoris.

Risk Factors: Depression anxiety, ADHD, personality disorders, psychotic disorders, smoking early in life, relative who smokes, and use of other substances.

Labs to Consider: Nonspecific.

Screening Scales

Tobacco, Alcohol, Prescription Medication, and Other Substance Use (TAPS)—It provides screening and brief assessment of commonly used drugs. It can be self-administered or administered by a clinician. Part one asks screens for use in the previous 12 months. If there is a positive answer, then part two screens for use in the past 3 months. If two or more answers are "yes" in part two, it is considered a positive screen with a 70% sensitivity for tobacco, alcohol, and marijuana.

The Alcohol, Smoking, and Substance Involvement Screening Test (ASSIST)—It is a clinician-driven screening assessment that screens for nine commonly abused substances. The first question screens for the drug and subsequent follow-up questions ask about frequency and attempts to cutback. The score is totaled, and based on that total, there is a chart for recommendations. This can be found on the World Health Organization's website.

Treatment

The US Preventive Services Task Force guidelines have recommended using the 5A approach to smoking cessation: **A**sk about tobacco use, **A**dvise quitting, **A**ssess readiness to quit, **A**ssist smokers ready to quit, and **A**rrange follow-up. Instructions on how to implement this routine into practice is available online. The best approach to cessation is a combination of psychosocial interventions and medication.

Non-pharmacologic Interventions

Cognitive Behavioral Therapy (CBT): It is a type of therapy that focuses on changing one's thoughts and behaviors to improve mood and functioning. It is a short-term, collaborative, goal-oriented therapy where the therapist helps the client identify negative thought patterns and behaviors and they develop ways to reconceptualize these thoughts and behaviors into something more positive.

Nicotine Anonymous: It is a 12-step program for people trying to stop their dependence on nicotine.

Pharmacologic Interventions

Bupropion SR (Wellbutrin SR)

Starting Dose: 150 mg PO daily.

Titration: Increase by 150 mg PO daily after 3 days.

Max Dose: 300 mg PO daily.

FDA Approval: MDD, seasonal affective disorder, nicotine addiction (standard release).

Common Side Effects: Dry mouth, GI upset, insomnia, dizziness, headache, agitation, anxiety, tremor, sweating, weight loss, anorexia, myalgia, tinnitus, rash, hypertension.

Rare: *Seizures, Stevens-Johnson syndrome, induction of mania, and activation of suicidal ideation in those under 24.*

Monitoring: PHQ-9.

PEARL: XL only requires once a day dosing, making it the preferred preparation. It can be given with other antidepressants to help with sexual side effects.

Contraindicated: Patients with current or prior diagnosis of bulimia or anorexia nervosa. Patients with a history of seizures. If a patient is abruptly quitting alcohol, sedative use, or anticonvulsant medication. If a patient has had a recent head injury or has a nervous system tumor [8].

Nicotine Transmucosal (Nicorette Gum)

First Cigarette More Than 30 min after Awakening: 2 mg by mouth every 1–2 h × 6 weeks, then every 2–4 h × 3 weeks, then every 4–8 h × 3 weeks.

First Cigarette Less Than 30 min after Awakening: 4 mg by mouth every 1–2 h × 6 weeks, then every 2–4 h × 3 weeks, then every 4–8 h × 3 weeks.

Max Dose: 24 mg.

FDA Approval: Nicotine dependence.

Common Side Effects: Withdrawal symptoms, palpitations, hypertension, nausea, hiccups, flatulence, cough, sore throat, paresthesia, arthralgia, URI symptoms.

Uncommon: *Nicotine dependence transference.*

Contraindications: Severe arrythmia, acute MI within last 2 weeks, worsening/severe angina.

PEARL: Avoid food or drink within 15 min before or after use [9].

Nicotine Transdermal (Nicoderm CQ)

Greater than 10 cigarettes per day: 21 mg transdermal daily × 6 weeks, then 14 mg/day × 2 weeks, then apply 7 mg patch daily × 2 weeks. Start on day 1 of quitting.

Less than 10 cigarettes per day: Apply 14 mg patch daily × 6 weeks, then apply 7 mg patch daily × 2 weeks. Start on day 1 of quitting.

FDA Approval: Nicotine addiction and dependence.

Common Side Effects: Local skin reaction and edema, rash, withdrawal symptoms, headache, palpitations, tachycardia, hypertension, nausea, hiccups, constipation, flatulence, diarrhea, paresthesia, arthralgia, chest discomfort, insomnia, and abnormal dreams.

Uncommon: *Nicotine dependence transference, hypersensitivity reaction.*

Contraindications: Severe arrythmia, acute MI within last 2 weeks, worsening/severe angina [10].

Other nicotine preparations include inhaler and lozenge.

Varenicline (Chantix)

Starting Dose: 0.5 mg PO daily.

Titration: After 3 days, increase to 0.5 mg PO BID, and after 4 days, increase to 1 mg PO BID.

Max Dose: 1 mg PO BID.

FDA Approval: Nicotine addiction and dependence.

Common Side Effects: Nausea, vomiting, constipation, flatulence, insomnia, headache, abnormal dreams,

Rare: Agitation, *depressed mood, suicidal ideation and behavior, seizures.*

PEARL: Take with meal and full glass of water. Pt should start treatment 1 week prior to quit date or quit smoking between 8 and 35 days of starting Chantix. Depression should be well controlled before starting [11].

References

1. Ewing. CAGE substance abuse screening tool; 1984. https://www.hopkinsmedicine.org/-/media/johns-hopkins-health-plans/documents/all_plans/cage-substance-screening-tool.pdf.

2. American Psychiatric Association. Substance-related and addictive disorders. In: Diagnostic and statistical manual of mental disorders (5th-TR). Washington, DC: American Psychiatric Association; 2022.
3. FOREST PHARMACEUTICALS, Inc. Campral; 2005. https://www.accessdata.fda.gov/drugsatfda_docs/label/2010/021431s013lbl.pdf.
4. Antabuse: Package insert; 2024. Drugs.com. https://www.drugs.com/pro/antabuse.html.
5. Duramed Pharmaceuticals Inc. Revia: prescriber highlights; 2013. https://www.accessdata.fda.gov/drugsatfda_docs/label/2013/018932s017lbl.pdf.
6. Alkermes. Vivitrol: highlights of prescribing information; 2010. https://www.accessdata.fda.gov/drugsatfda_docs/label/2010/021897s015lbl.pdf.
7. Janssen Pharmaceuticals, Inc. Topamax: highlights of prescribing information; 2009. https://www.accessdata.fda.gov/drugsatfda_docs/label/2017/020505s057_020844s048lbl.pdf.
8. GlaxoSmithKline. Wellbutrin SR: prescribing information; 2009. https://www.accessdata.fda.gov/drugsatfda_docs/label/2009/020358s046s047lbl.pdf.
9. Nicorette gum (nicotine gum) dosing, indications, interactions, adverse effects, and more; 2024. https://reference.medscape.com/drug/nicorette-gum-nicotine-gum-999317#0.
10. GlaxoSmithKline Consumer Healthcare, LP. Nicoderm CQ: prescribing information; 2006. https://www.accessdata.fda.gov/drugsatfda_docs/label/2006/020165s023lbl.pdf.
11. Pfizer Labs. Chantix: highlights of prescribing information; 2019. https://www.pfizermedicalinformation.com/chantix/highlights.

Schizophrenia

9

Contents

Schizophrenia

Schizophrenia is a chronic psychiatric illness that is hallmarked by recurrent psychosis. It is a syndrome that involves four symptom domains. Positive symptoms include hallucinations (auditory, visual, somatic, olfactory, or gustatory), delusions, and/or disorganization. Negative symptoms include blunted affect, alogia, avolition, apathy, and asociality. Impairments in cognition are also prevalent, such as decreased processing speed, decreased attention and working memory, and decreased social cognition. The last domain affects the mood and causes anxiety in the patient.

B. Floyd, T. Kane, *The Clinician's Guide to Common Psychiatric Disorders*, https://doi.org/10.1007/978-3-031-67958-2_9

Diagnosing and Monitoring

DSM-5-TR

Per the DSM-5-TR, a schizophrenia diagnosis needs two of the following symptoms, and one of them must be from the bolded list:

- **Delusions**
- **Hallucinations**
- **Disorganized speech**
- Grossly disorganized or catatonic behavior
- Negative symptoms

Symptoms have to be present for at least 1 month or less if successfully treated. There also needs to be a significant decrease in level of functioning from the individual such as work or ability to care for self. Signs of the disturbance must be present for at least 6 months (including the 1 month of symptoms). The disturbance cannot be attributed to a medical condition or a substance, and both bipolar and schizoaffective disorders have never been diagnosed. For a more complete list of requirements, see the DSM-5-TR on pages 113–114[1, pp. 113–114].

Differential Diagnosis: Bipolar 1 with psychotic features, delusional disorder, schizoaffective, brief psychotic disorder, certain personality disorders, drug/medication-induced psychosis, psychosis secondary to organic causes, and psychotic depression.

Risk Factors: First-degree relative with schizophrenia, prenatal malnutrition, exposure to certain viruses prenatal, living in an urban area, immigration, advanced paternal age, and obstetrical complications.

Labs to Consider: Nonspecific but may want baseline CBC, CMP, A1c, lipid panel for monitoring. Drugs of abuse urine screen if indicated.

Screening Scales

Scale for Assessment of Positive Symptoms (SAPS): It is used in conjunction with the SANS. It consists of a total of 34 items. It measures positive symptoms such as hallucinations, delusions, bizarre behavior, and thought disorder. Takes about 30 min to complete and is clinician driven.

Scale for the Assessment of Negative Symptoms (SANS): It is used in conjunction with the SAPS. It consists of a total of 19 items incorporating 5 scales: Affective flattening or blunting, alogia, avolition-apathy, anhedonia-asociality, and inattention. The time required varies and it is clinician rated.

Positive and Negative Syndrome Scale (PANSS): **It is the** gold standard for measuring effectiveness of schizophrenia treatment. Generally, it takes 30–40 min to complete by a trained clinician. Some critics consider the tool outdated.

Treatment

First-line treatment for schizophrenia is medication, more specifically second-generation antipsychotics. While the main goal of treatment is complete remission of psychotic symptoms, a large portion of patients will have residual symptoms. The goal at this point is to gain a level of control that does not interfere with everyday life.

There is utility in psychotherapy once the patient is no longer acutely psychotic. Psychotherapies that show benefit with patients with schizophrenia are cognitive behavioral therapy, group therapy/support groups, assertive community treatment, milieu therapy, and client/family education.

Non-pharmacologic Interventions

Cognitive Behavioral Therapy: It is a type of therapy that focuses on changing one's thoughts and behaviors to improve mood and functioning. It is a short-term, collaborative, goal-oriented therapy where the therapist helps the client identify negative thought patterns and behaviors, and they develop ways to reconceptualize these thoughts and behaviors into something more positive.

Assertive Community Treatment: It is a mental health delivery system for those with severe mental illness. It offers case management, treatment, rehabilitation, and support services to enable patients to live a life as independently as possible.

Milieu Therapy: It is a therapy that uses a person's surroundings to encourage healthier ways of thinking and behaving while avoiding self-destructive behavior. It is used mostly in group settings.

Hospitalization

While laws vary by state, it is prudent to ensure the safety of your patient and those around them. If a person is an immediate threat to themselves (suicidal ideation) or others (homicidal ideations), it is generally considered reason enough to send patient for hospitalization. Also, if the patient is so psychotic that they cannot meet their basic needs (showering, preparing/eating meals), then it may warrant hospitalization.

Managing a schizophrenic patient can be outside of the scope of a general practitioner. It is recommended to make an early referral to a psychiatric specialist if there is suspicion of schizophrenia. The following list of medications is a good starting point, and Clozaril is intentionally left out as the provider needs to be part of the REMS program to prescribe it. It may make sense to prescribe one of the other medications while awaiting expert consultation. If the patient is at risk to themselves or others, immediate referral to the Emergency Department is warranted.

First-Line Medications

Aripiprazole (Abilify)

Starting Dose: 15 mg PO daily.

Titration: Increase by 5–10 mg PO daily every week.

Max Dose: 30 mg PO daily.

FDA Approval: Depression adjunct, schizophrenia, bipolar maintenance, acute mania/mixed mood.

Common Side Effects: Dizziness, insomnia, akathisia, activation, nausea, vomiting, headache, orthostatic hypotension, and tardive dyskinesia.

Monitoring: PHQ-9, BMI every 3 months, lipid panel, and A1c annually. AIMS score every 3–6 months.

Pearl: Injectable form available.

Rare: *Impulse control problems (gambling), hyperglycemia, neuroleptic malignant syndrome (NMS), and seizures.*

Black Box Warning: Elderly dementia patients who take Abilify have a higher risk of death. Use may increase suicidal thoughts in children, adolescents, and young adults [2].

Asenapine (Saphris)

Starting Dose: 10 mg sublingual BID (20 mg/day).

Titration: Reduce to 5 mg sublingual BID (10 mg/day) if adverse effects.

Max Dose: 20 mg/day.

FDA Approval: Schizophrenia, mania/mixed mania, and bipolar maintenance.

Common Side Effects: Increased risk for diabetes and dyslipidemia, dizziness, sedation, dry mouth, constipation, weight gain, edema, musculoskeletal pain, orthostatic hypotension, tardive dyskinesia.

Uncommon: *Type 1 hypersensitivity reactions, hyperglycemia, rare neuroleptic malignant syndrome, rare seizures.*

Monitoring: PHQ-9, BMI every 3 months, lipid panel, and A1c annually. Waist circumference, blood pressure, fasting plasma glucose, and fasting lipid profile prior to start, within 3 months, and then annually.

Contraindications: Severe hepatic impairment.

Black Box Warning: Elderly dementia patients who take Saphris have a higher risk of death. Use may increase suicidal thoughts in children, adolescents, and young adults (24 and younger) [3].

Cariprazine (Vraylar)

Starting Dose: 1.5 mg PO daily.

Titration: 1.5 mg daily.

Max Dose: 6 mg. Recommended range: 3–6 mg.

FDA Approval: Schizophrenia acute and maintenance, acute mania/mixed mood, bipolar 1 (depression).

Common Side Effects: Akathisia, EPS, restlessness, GI distress, sedation, tardive dyskinesia.

Rare: *Hyperglycemia, neuroleptic malignant syndrome, and seizures.*

Monitoring: BMI monthly × 3 months then every 3 months. Blood pressure, fasting plasma glucose, fasting lipid panel within 3 months and then monthly. More often if at risk for metabolic syndrome.

Caveats: Side effects may develop weeks later due to long half-life.

Black Box Warning: Elderly dementia patients who take Abilify have a higher risk of death. Use may increase suicidal thoughts in children, adolescents, and young adults [4].

Lumateperone (Caplyta)

Starting Dose: 42 mg.

Titration: None needed.

Max 42 mg.

FDA Approval: Schizophrenia, bipolar depression.

Common Side Effects: Sedation, dry mouth, tardive dyskinesia.

Uncommon: *Hyperglycemia, neuroleptic malignant syndrome, seizures.*

Monitoring: BMI monthly × 3 months then every 3 months. Blood pressure, fasting plasma glucose, fasting lipid panel within 3 months and then monthly. More often if at risk for metabolic syndrome.

Caveats: Not known for metabolic side effects.

Black Box Warning: Elderly dementia patients who take Abilify have a higher risk of death. Use may increase suicidal thoughts in children, adolescents, and young adults [5].

Lurasidone (Latuda)

Starting Dose: 40 mg PO daily with the largest meal.

Titration: Increase by 20–40 mg PO daily every week.

Max Dose: 160 mg PO daily.

FDA Approval: Schizophrenia, bipolar depression.

Common Side Effects: Sedation, akathisia, nausea, hyperprolactinemia, increased risk of diabetes and dyslipidemia, tardive dyskinesia.

Uncommon: *Tachycardia/first-degree AV block, hyperglycemia (ketoacidosis), NMS, seizures.*

Monitoring: BMI monthly × 3 months then every 3 months. Blood pressure, fasting plasma glucose, fasting lipid panel within 3 months and then monthly. More often if at risk for metabolic syndrome.

Caveats: Give with >350 calories. Used in depressed state, watch for s/s of mania.

Contraindications: Taking a strong CYP 3A4 inhibitor/inducer (ketoconazole, rifampin), history of angioedema.

Black Box Warning: Elderly dementia patients who take Abilify have a higher risk of death. Use may increase suicidal thoughts in children, adolescents, and young adults [6].

Olanzapine (Zyprexa)

Starting Dose: 5–10 mg.

Titration: 5 mg/day once a week.

Max Dose: 20 mg/day.

FDA Approval: Schizophrenia, mania/mixed mania, bipolar maintenance, acute agitation associated with bipolar 1 mania.

Common Side Effects: Increased risk for diabetes and dyslipidemia, dizziness, sedation, dry mouth, constipation, weight gain, edema, musculoskeletal pain, orthostatic hypotension, tardive dyskinesia.

Rare: *DRESS, hyperglycemia (ketoacidosis), NMS, seizures.*

Monitoring: GAD-7, BMI every 3 months, lipid panel, and A1c annually. Waist circumference, blood pressure, fasting plasma glucose, and fasting lipid profile prior to start, within 3 months, and then annually. AIMS score every 3–6 months.

Pearl: Patient maybe given prn in ½ tablets of 2.5 mg tablets.

Contraindications: Risk of angle-closure glaucoma, unstable cardiac condition.

Black Box Warning: Elderly dementia patients who take Zyprexa have a higher risk of death. Use may increase suicidal thoughts in children, adolescents, and young adults (24 and younger) [7].

Olanzapine-Fluoxetine (Symbyax)

Starting Dose: 6 mg/25 mg mg PO daily.

Titration: Increase by 3 mg of olanzapine or 25 mg of fluoxetine.

Max Dose: 18 mg/75 mg mg PO daily.

FDA Approval: Treatment-resistant depression, schizophrenia, bipolar maintenance, bipolar depression.

Common Side Effects: Increased risk of diabetes and dyslipidemia, dizziness, sedation, dry mouth, constipation, weight gain, edema, musculoskeletal pain, orthostatic hypotension, tardive dyskinesia.

Rare: *DRESS, hyperglycemia, neuroleptic malignant syndrome, seizures.*

Monitoring: PHQ-9, BMI every 3 months, lipid panel, and A1c annually. Waist circumference, blood pressure, fasting plasma glucose, and fasting lipid profile prior to start, within 3 months, and then annually. AIMS score every 3–6 months.

Contraindications: Known risk of angle-closure glaucoma or unstable cardiac condition.

Black Box Warning: Elderly dementia patients who take Symbyax have a higher risk of death. Use may increase suicidal thoughts in children, adolescents, and young adults (24 and younger) [8].

Quetiapine (Seroquel)

Starting Dose: 50 mg PO BID.

Titration: 100 mg/day. Once at 400 mg/day, may increase by 200 mg/day.

Max Dose: 800 mg PO daily.

FDA Approval: MDD, bipolar depression, bipolar maintenance, schizophrenia.

Common Side Effects: GI upset, sexual dysfunction, insomnia, agitation, sedation, dizziness, urinary retention, headache, weight loss, myalgia, sweating, anorexia, hypertension, and nausea better in 3–5 days.

Rare: *Neuroleptic malignant syndrome, seizures.*

Monitoring: PHQ-9, BMI every 3 months, lipid panel, and A1c annually. Waist circumference, blood pressure, fasting plasma glucose, and fasting lipid profile prior to start, within 3 months, and then annually. AIMS score every 3–6 months.

Pearl: It is known for its sedating properties; it could be useful as an insomnia adjunct in doses up to 100 mg.

Black Box Warning: Elderly dementia patients who take Seroquel have a higher risk of death. Use may increase suicidal thoughts in children, adolescents, and young adults (24 and younger) [9, 10].

Quetiapine XR (Seroquel XR)

Starting Dose: 300 mg PO nightly.

Titration: Increase by 300 mg PO nightly.

Max Dose: Usually 800 mg PO nightly for depression.

FDA Approval: MDD, bipolar depression, bipolar maintenance, schizophrenia.

Common Side Effects: GI upset, sexual dysfunction, insomnia, agitation, sedation, dizziness, urinary retention, headache, weight loss, myalgia, sweating, anorexia, hypertension, and nausea better in 3–5 days.

Rare: *Neuroleptic malignant syndrome, seizures.*

Monitoring: PHQ-9, BMI every 3 months, lipid panel, and A1c annually. Waist circumference, blood pressure, fasting plasma glucose, and fasting lipid profile prior to start, within 3 months, and then annually. AIMS score every 3–6 months.

Pearl: It is known for its sedating properties; it could be useful as an insomnia adjunct in doses up to 100 mg.

Black Box Warning: Elderly dementia patients who take Seroquel have a higher risk of death. Use may increase suicidal thoughts in children, adolescents, and young adults (24 and younger) [9, 10].

Risperidone (Risperdal)

Starting Dose: 0.5 mg PO BID (1 mg/day).

Titration: Increase by 1 mg/day, every day.

Max Dose: 16 mg/day.

FDA Approval: Schizophrenia, acute mania/mixed mania, autism-related irritability in children, and bipolar maintenance.

Common Side Effects: Increased risk for diabetes and dyslipidemia, drug-induced parkinsonism, hyperprolactinemia, dizziness, insomnia, anxiety, sedation, GI distress, weight gain, sexual dysfunction, tardive dyskinesia, and orthostatic hypotension.

Uncommon/Rare: *Hyperglycemia, neuroleptic malignant syndrome, seizures.*

Monitoring: PHQ-9, BMI every 3 months, lipid panel, and A1c annually. Waist circumference, blood pressure, fasting plasma glucose, and fasting lipid profile prior to start, within 3 months, and then annually.

Black Box Warning: Elderly dementia patients who take Zyprexa have a higher risk of death. Use may increase suicidal thoughts in children, adolescents, and young adults (24 and younger) [11].

References

1. American Psychiatric Association. Schizophrenia spectrum and other psychotic disorders. In: Diagnostic and statistical manual of mental disorders (5th-TR). Washington, DC: American Psychiatric Association; 2022.
2. Otsuka American Pharmaceutical, Inc. Abilify: highlights of prescribing information; 2022. https://www.otsuka-us.com/sites/g/files/qhldwo7626/files/media/static/Abilify-PI.pdf.
3. Merck, Sharp & Dohme B. V. Saphris: highlights of prescribing information; 2017. https://www.accessdata.fda.gov/drugsatfda_docs/label/2017/022117s020s021lbl.pdf.
4. Forest Laboratories Holdings Ltd. Vraylar: highlights of prescribing information; 2022. https://www.rxabbvie.com/pdf/vraylar_pi.pdf.
5. Intracellular Therapies. Caplyta: highlights of prescribing information; 2023. https://www.intracellulartherapies.com/docs/caplyta_pi.pdf.
6. Sunovion Pharmaceuticals Inc. Latuda: highlights of prescribing information; 2013. https://www.accessdata.fda.gov/drugsatfda_docs/label/2013/200603lbls10s11.pdf.
7. Eli Lilly and Company. Zyprexa: highlights of prescribing information; 2021. https://pi.lilly.com/us/zyprexa-pi.pdf.
8. Eli Lilly and Company. Symbyax: highlights of prescribing information; 2023. https://pi.lilly.com/us/symbyax-pi.pdf.
9. AstraZeneca Pharmaceuticals LP. Seroquel: highlights of prescribing information; 2009. https://www.accessdata.fda.gov/drugsatfda_docs/label/2009/020639s045s046lbl.pdf.
10. AstraZeneca Pharmaceuticals LP. Seroquel XR: highlights of prescribing information; 2009. https://www.accessdata.fda.gov/drugsatfda_docs/label/2009/022047s011s016s017s019s022lbl.pdf.
11. Janssen Pharmaceutical Companies. Risperdal: highlights of prescribing information; 2007. https://www.accessdata.fda.gov/drugsatfda_docs/label/2019/020272s082,020588s070,021444s056lbl.pdf.

Eating Disorders

10

Contents

B. Floyd, T. Kane, *The Clinician's Guide to Common Psychiatric Disorders*, https://doi.org/10.1007/978-3-031-67958-2_10

Anorexia Nervosa

Anorexia Nervosa is an eating disorder characterized by an extreme preoccupation with thinness. Many people with anorexia tie their self-worth to their ability to be thin. Several key features include extremely low body weight, intense fear of gaining weight, distorted perception of weight, extreme efforts to control weight, and maladaptive coping mechanisms.

Diagnosing and Monitoring

Mnemonic: Anorexia: Anorexic patients try to get **RID** of their weight.

R—**Restriction** of intake leading to significantly low body weight
I—**Intense** fear of weight gain
D—**Disturbance** in perception of one's weight or body image [1]

DSM-5-TR

The DSM-5-TR described anorexia nervosa as a "restriction of energy intake relative to requirements, leading to a significantly low body weight in the context of age, sex, developmental trajectory, and physical health. Significantly low weight is defined as a weight that is less than minimally normal or, for children and adolescents, less than that minimally expected."

The patient must have an overwhelming fear of becoming overweight, gaining weight, or behaviors that interfere with weight gain, even though they are significantly underweight. Pt also must have a disturbance in how their body shape is experienced or persistent lack of recognition or underplaying of the seriousness of their low body weight. You can specify if it is restricting type which is using restrictive methods such as fasting, heavy dieting, or heavy exercise for the past 3 months. Binge-eating/purging type has the patient binge-eat and then purge through vomiting, enemas, or laxatives within the past 3 months. It is categorized as mild, moderate, or severe based on BMI. For a more complete list of requirements, see the DSM-5-TR on page 381 [2, p. 381].

Differential Diagnosis: Avoidant/restrictive food intake disorder, bulimia nervosa, MDD, social anxiety disorder, substance use disorder.

Risk Factors: Genetic loading, first-degree relative with eating disorders, mood disorders, rigid perfectionism, and substance abuse disorders.

Vital Signs: Initial physical exam should include temperature, heart rate, blood pressure, orthostatic pulse, orthostatic blood pressure, height, weight, and BMI [3].

Labs to Consider: Should include CBC and CMP. EKG in patients with a restrictive eating disorder, severe purging, or those taking medications known to prolong QTc.

Screening Scales

Eating Disorder Diagnostic Scale: It is a brief (22 items) self-report questionnaire/scale to help diagnose eating disorders such as anorexia nervosa, bulimia nervosa, and binge-eating disorder. A more updated version is available to align with DSM-5-TR criteria [4].

SCOFF Screening Questionnaire: It is developed in the United Kingdom but can be adaptable in the United States with slight modifications. Sensitivity is 100% and specificity is 90% for anorexia nervosa. It is not a diagnostic tool, but two positive responses are strong indicators of an eating disorder.

Do you make yourself ***S***ick (induce vomiting) because you feel uncomfortably full?
Do you worry you have lost ***C***ontrol over how much you eat?
Have you recently lost more than ***O***ne stone [*approximately fifteen pounds*] in a 3-month period?
Do you believe yourself to be ***F***at when others say you are too thin?
Would you say that ***F***ood dominates your life [5]?

Treatment

Patients who require nutritional rehabilitation and weight restoration should have individualized goals for weekly weight gain and target weight.

Patients should be treated with an eating disorder focused psychotherapy, which should normalize eating and weight control behaviors, restoring weight, and addressing psychological aspects of the disorder.

Adolescents that have an involved caregiver should be treated with an eating disorder-focused family-based treatment which should include caregiver education.

There are no FDA-approved pharmacological interventions for anorexia nervosa [3].

Hospitalization Criteria

- "To avert potentially irreversible effects on physical growth and development, many children and adolescents require inpatient medical treatment, even when weight loss, although rapid, has not been as severe as that suggesting a need for hospitalization in adult patients.
- Hospitalization should occur before the onset of medical instability as manifested by abnormalities in vital signs:
  - Orthostatic hypotension with an increase in pulse of 20 bpm
  - Drop in standing blood pressure of 20 mmHg
  - Bradycardia <40 bpm
  - Tachycardia >110 bpm
  - Inability to sustain core body temperature" (Anorexia [6])

Bulimia Nervosa

Bulimia nervosa is an eating disorder that is characterized by eating large quantities of food at one time (binging) followed by extreme fasting or self-induced vomiting (purging) to try to compensate for excessive calories. Those with bulimia tend to have excessive concern with weight and body shape. Purging may lead to dehydration, digestive distress, esophageal tears, heart damage, heartburn, and tooth decay. Binging may also lead to diabetes, heart disease, high blood pressure, liver disease, and sleep problems.

DSM-5-TR

The DSM-5-TR describes bulimia nervosa as binge-eating episodes followed by purging activities. A binge-eating episode is characterized by eating a larger than normal amount of food that most individuals would eat in a similar time period AND the patient feels a lack of control of the binging during the episode. Binging is inappropriate compensatory behaviors such as vomiting, misusing laxatives, medications, or excessive fasting in order to prevent weight gain. This usually happens on average at least once a week for 3 months, and patient's self-evaluation is unduly influenced by body shape. This occurs outside of an anorexia diagnosis. Severity is based on number of compensatory occurring in a week. For a more complete list of diagnostic criteria, see the DSM-5-TR on page 387 [2, p. 387].

Differential Diagnosis: Anorexia nervosa, body dysmorphic disorder, depression, gastric outlet obstruction, obsessive-compulsive disorder.

Risk Factors: Genetic loading, first degree relative with eating disorders, mood disorders, rigid perfectionism, and substance abuse disorders.

Vital Signs: Initial physical exam should include temperature, heart rate, blood pressure, orthostatic pulse, orthostatic blood pressure, height, weight, and BMI [3].

Labs to Consider: Should include CBC and CMP. EKG in patients with a restrictive eating disorder, severe purging, or those taking medications known to prolong QTc.

Screening Scales

Eating Disorder Diagnostic Scale: It is a brief (22 items) self-report questionnaire/scale to help diagnose eating disorders such as anorexia nervosa, bulimia nervosa, and binge-eating disorder.

A more updated version is available to align with DSM-5-TR criteria [4].

SCOFF Screening Questionnaire: It is developed in the United Kingdom but can be adaptable in the United States with slight modifications. Sensitivity is 100% and specificity is 90% for anorexia nervosa. It is not a diagnostic tool, but two positive responses are strong indicators of an eating disorder.

Do you make yourself ***S***ick (induce vomiting) because you feel uncomfortably full?
Do you worry you have lost ***C***ontrol over how much you eat?
Have you recently lost more than ***O***ne stone [*approximately fifteen pounds*] in a 3-month period?
Do you believe yourself to be ***F***at when others say you are too thin?
Would you say that ***F***ood dominates your life [5]?

Treatment

Adults with bulimia nervosa should be treated with eating disorder-focused cognitive behavioral therapy, and a serotonin reuptake inhibitor may also be prescribed either initially or if there is minimal to no response to psychotherapy alone by 6 weeks of treatment.

Adolescents with bulimia nervosa who have an involved caregiver should be treated with eating disorder-focused family-based treatment [3].

First-Line Medication

Fluoxetine (Prozac)

Starting Dose: 20 mg PO daily. 10 mg PO daily can be used in elderly.
Titration: Increase by 20 mg PO daily every week. Wait for 4–6 weeks for the response when initializing therapy.

Max Dose: 80 mg PO daily.
FDA Approval: MDD (8 and older), OCD (7 and older), PMDD, **bulimia**, and panic disorder.
Common Side Effects: GI upset, sexual dysfunction, insomnia, agitation, headache, and nausea better in 3–5 days.
Monitoring: PHQ-9, ECG if QT prolongation. Height and weight on children.
Pearl: No need to taper due to long half-life [7].

Prozac is the only SSRI with FDA approval to treat bulimia nervosa. Other SSRIs will be considered off-label.

Binge-Eating Disorder

Binge-eating disorder (BED) is an eating disorder characterized by a person that eats excessively large quantities of food at one time. Unlike bulimia, there is not an attempt to get rid of excessive calories so there is no fasting or purging behaviors. Most people with BED are overweight. They are also at risk for diabetes, heart disease, high blood pressure, liver disease, and sleep problems.

DSM-5-TR

The DSM-5-TR describes binge-eating as an episode that is characterized by eating a larger than normal amount of food that most individuals would eat in a similar time period AND the patient feels a lack of control of the binging during the episode. The binging episodes are associated with three of the following:

1. Eating much more rapidly than normal
2. Eating until feeling uncomfortably full
3. Eating large amounts of food when not feeling physically hungry
4. Eating alone because of feeling embarrassed by how much one is eating
5. Feeling disgusted with oneself, depressed, or very guilty afterward

This behavior occurs at least once a week for 3 months and is not associated with anorexia of bulimia. There is also marked distress about the binge-eating. It is also classified by severity based on number of binging episodes per week. For more complete diagnostic criteria, see the DSM-5-TR on page 392 [2, p. 392].

Differential Diagnosis: Bulimia nervosa, mood disorders, anxiety disorders, obesity, borderline personality disorder.

Screening Scales

Eating Disorder Diagnostic Scale: It is a brief (22 items) self-report questionnaire/scale to help diagnose eating disorders such as anorexia nervosa, bulimia nervosa, and binge-eating disorder. A more updated version is available to align with DSM-5-TR criteria [4].

SCOFF Screening Questionnaire: It is developed in the United Kingdom but can be adaptable in the United States with slight modifications. Sensitivity is 100% and specificity is 90% for anorexia nervosa. It is not a diagnostic tool, but two positive responses are strong indicators of an eating disorder.

Do you make yourself ***S***ick (induce vomiting) because you feel uncomfortably full?
Do you worry you have lost ***C***ontrol over how much you eat?
Have you recently lost more than ***O***ne stone [*approximately fifteen pounds*] in a 3-month period?
Do you believe yourself to be ***F***at when others say you are too thin?
Would you say that ***F***ood dominates your life [5]?

Risk Factors: Genetic loading, first-degree relative with eating disorders, mood disorders, and substance abuse disorders.

Vital Signs: Initial physical exam should include temperature, heart rate, blood pressure, orthostatic pulse, orthostatic blood pressure, height, weight, and BMI [3].

Labs to Consider: Should include CBC and CMP. EKG in patients with a restrictive eating disorder, severe purging, or those taking medications known to prolong QTc.

Treatment

Adults with binge-eating disorder should be treated with eating disorder-focused cognitive behavioral therapy or interpersonal therapy, in either group or individual formats [3].

Patients who prefer medication or who have not responded to psychotherapy alone should be treated with either an antidepressant or Vyvanse.

First-Line Medication

Lisdexamfetamine (Vyvanse)

Starting Dose: 30 mg PO daily.
Titration: Increase 20 mg PO daily every week.
Max Dose: 70 mg/day.
FDA Approval: ADHD ages 6 and up. **Binge-eating disorder**.
Common Side Effects: Fatigue, sleepiness, insomnia, irritability, headache, decreased appetite, nausea, vomiting, dry mouth, constipation, increased heart rate and blood pressure, hypomania.
Monitoring: Blood pressure at initiation, after dose increase, and periodically throughout treatment.
Contraindications: Taking MAOI inhibitor, history of pheochromocytoma, angle-closure glaucoma, hyperthyroidism, and severe cardiovascular disorder.
Pearl: Taper to avoid withdrawal effects [8].

SSRIs are used off-label. When in doubt, refer out.

References

1. Caplan J, Stern T. Mnemonics in a mnutshell: 32 aids to psychiatric diagnosis. Curr Psychiatr Ther. 2008;7(10):27–33.
2. American Psychiatric Association. Feeding and eating disorders. In: Diagnostic and statistical manual of mental disorders (5th-TR). Washington, DC: American Psychiatric Association; 2022.
3. Crone C, Fochtmann J, Attia E, Boland R, Escobar J, Fornari V, Golden N, Guarda A, Jackson-Triche M, Manzo L, Mascolo M, Pierce K, Riddle M, Seritan A, Uniacke B, Zucker N. The American Psychiatric Association Practice Guideline for treatment of patients with eating disorders; 2022. Psychiatry.org. https://www.psychiatry.org/getmedia/97405f0d-1bd4-43d0-abdd-c013fcd8686d/APA-Eating-Disorders-Practice-Guideline-Under-Copyediting.pdf.
4. Bohon C, Stice E. Eating disorder diagnostic scale. In: Wade T, editor. Encyclopedia of feeding and eating disorders. Singapore: Springer; 2015. https://doi.org/10.1007/978-981-287-087-2_109-1.
5. Cowden S. The SCOFF Questionnaire Screens for Eating Disorders [Review of The SCOFF Questionnaire Screens for Eating Disorders]; 2022, February 9. VeryWellMind. https://www.verywellmind.com/the-scoff-questionnaire-1138316.
6. Anorexia Nervosa. PsychDB; 2021, May 18. https://www.psychdb.com/eating-disorders/anorexia#google_vignette.
7. Eli Lilly and Company. Prozac: highlights of prescribing information; 1987. https://pi.lilly.com/us/prozac.pdf.
8. Takeda Pharmaceutical Company. Vyvanse: highlights of prescribing information; 2021. https://www.accessdata.fda.gov/drugsatfda_docs/label/2021/021977s046,208510s003lbl.pdf.

Appendix A

Antidepressants/Anxiolytics

Bupropion XL (Wellbutrin XL)—Norepinephrine and Dopamine Reuptake Inhibitor (NDRI)

Starting Dose: 150 mg PO daily.

Titration: Increase by 150 mg PO daily. Wait 4–6 weeks for response when initializing therapy.

Max Dose: 450 mg PO daily.

FDA Approval: MDD, seasonal affective disorder, nicotine addiction (standard release).

Common Side Effects: Dry mouth, constipation, GI upset, insomnia, dizziness, headache, agitation, anxiety, tremor, sweating, weight loss, anorexia, myalgia, tinnitus, rash, and hypertension.

Rare: *Seizures, Stevens-Johnson syndrome has been reported, induction of mania, and activation of suicidal ideation in those under 24.*

Monitoring: PHQ-9 and blood pressure.

Pearl: XL only requires once a day dosing, making it the preferred preparation. Can be given with other antidepressants to help with sexual side effects.

Contraindicated: Patients with current or prior diagnosis of bulimia or anorexia nervosa. Patients with a history of seizures. If a patient is abruptly quitting alcohol, sedative use, or anticon-

B. Floyd, T. Kane, *The Clinician's Guide to Common Psychiatric Disorders*, https://doi.org/10.1007/978-3-031-67958-2

vulsant medication. If a patient has had a recent head injury or has a nervous system tumor. If a patient is taking an MAO-I or Thioridazine.

Buspirone (Buspar)

Starting Dose: 5 mg PO daily.

Titration: Increase to 5 mg PO BID after 5–7 days. BID dosing is usually easiest.

Max Dose: 60 mg/day.

FDA Approval: Management of anxiety disorders.

Common Side Effects: Dizziness, nervousness, sedation, GI issues, headache, agitation.

Rare: *Cardiac symptoms.*

Monitoring: GAD-7.

Pearl: Should be taken every day scheduled for best efficacy, should not be used as needed.

Contraindication: Taking an MAO-I.

Citalopram (Celexa)

Starting Dose: 20 mg PO daily. Can use 10 mg PO daily in elderly.

Titration: Increase to 40 mg PO daily—wait 4–6 weeks for response when initializing therapy.

Max Dose: 40 mg PO daily.

FDA Approval: Depression.

Common Side Effects: GI upset, sexual dysfunction, agitation, headache, bruising, and nausea (better in 3–5 days).

Rare: *Seizures, hyponatremia, induction of mania, QTc prolongation, Serotonin Syndrome, bleeding, SIADH, and activation of suicidal ideation in those under 24.*

Monitoring: PHQ-9, ECG (if high risk or multiple QT prolonging medications), height and weight on children.

Contraindications: Taking MAO-I, pimozide, and known hypersensitivity to citalopram. Avoid in untreated Angle-Closure Glaucoma.

Black Box Warning: May increase suicidal thoughts in children, adolescents, and young adults (24 and younger).

Clomipramine (Anafranil)

Starting Dose: 25 mg PO daily.

Titration: Increase (as tolerated) to get to 100 mg PO daily at week 2.

Max Dose: 250 mg PO daily.

FDA Approval: Obsessive Compulsive Disorder.

Common Side Effects: Blurred vision, constipation, dry mouth, weight gain, dizziness, sedation, fatigue, rash, GI upset, sexual dysfunction, sweating, insomnia, agitation, headache, nausea better in 3–5 days.

Rare: *Seizures, paralytic ileus, orthostatic hypotension, QTc prolongation, hepatic failure, increased intraocular pressure, hyponatremia, induction of mania, and activation of suicidal ideation in those under 24.*

Monitoring: EKG if over 50. Associated with weight gain, determine BMI and metabolic risk before starting.

Pearl: Usually given with food while titrating. Once at established dose it is given at night to avoid daytime sedation.

Contraindications: Taking MAO-I, thioridazine, pimozide, or tamoxifen. Recovering from Myocardial Infarction. History of QTc prolongation, recent MI, or uncompensated heart failure.

Desvenlafaxine (Pristiq)

Starting Dose: 50 mg PO daily.

Titration: Increase by 50 mg PO daily. Wait 4–6 weeks for response when initializing therapy.

Max Dose: 400 mg PO daily.

FDA Approval: MDD.

Common Side Effects: Increased blood pressure, GI upset, sexual dysfunction, insomnia, dizziness, agitation, anxiety, sweating, headache, and nausea (better in 3–5 days).

Rare: *Seizures, hyponatremia, induction of mania, serotonin syndrome, SIADH, and activation of suicidal ideation in those under 24.*

Monitoring: PHQ-9 and blood pressure at each visit.

Pearl: Higher doses are associated with more side effects.

Contraindications: Uncontrolled angle-closure glaucoma or taking an MAO-I.

Black Box Warning: May increase suicidal thoughts in children, adolescents, and young adults (24 and younger).

Dextromethorphan/Bupropion (Auvelity)—NDRI/NMDA Receptor Antagonist

Starting Dose: 45–105 mg PO daily.

Titration: Take 1 PO daily × 3 days and then take 1 PO twice daily. Take at least 8 h apart.

Max Dose: 90–210 mg PO daily.

FDA Approval: Major Depressive Disorder.

Common Side Effects: Dizziness, headache, somnolence, diarrhea, dry mouth, hyperhidrosis and sexual dysfunction.

Rare: *Increased blood pressure, seizures, serotonin syndrome, psychosis, and induction of mania.*

Monitoring: PHQ-9 and blood pressure.

Pearl: Newest antidepressant on the market. Works NMDA receptors and can alleviate depression in a 1 week compared to 4–6 weeks of traditional antidepressants.

Contraindicated: Patients with current or prior diagnosis of bulimia or anorexia nervosa. Patients with a history of seizures. If a patient is abruptly quitting alcohol, sedative use, or anticonvulsant medication. If a patient has had a recent head injury or has a nervous system tumor. Taking a MAO-I.

Black Box Warning: May increase suicidal thoughts in children, adolescents, and young adults (24 and younger).

Duloxetine (Cymbalta)

Starting Dose: 40 mg PO daily.

Titration: Increase by 20 mg PO daily first titration. Wait 4–6 weeks for response when initializing therapy. Then may increase by 30 mg PO daily.

Max Dose: 120 mg PO daily.

FDA Approval: MDD, diabetic peripheral neuropathy, fibromyalgia, GAD, chronic musculoskeletal pain.

Common Side Effects: Increased blood pressure, GI upset, sexual dysfunction, insomnia, agitation, fatigue, dry mouth, sedation, sweating, dizziness, urinary retention, headache, blurred vision, and nausea (better in 3–5 days).

Rare: *Seizures, hyponatremia, induction of mania, possible hepatotoxicity, orthostatic hypotension, serotonin syndrome, bleeding, SIADH, and activation of suicidal ideation in those under 24.*

Monitoring: PHQ-9 and blood pressure at each visit.

PEARL: May get benefit of pain reduction on 30 mg dose. Should avoid with hepatic insufficiency.

Contraindications: Untreated angle-closure glaucoma, substantial alcohol use, taking an MAO-I, taking thioridazine.

Black Box Warning: May increase suicidal thoughts in children, adolescents, and young adults (24 and younger).

Escitalopram (Lexapro)

Starting Dose: 10 mg PO daily. Can use 5 mg PO daily in elderly.

Titration: Increase by 5–10 mg PO daily after 1 week. Wait 4–6 weeks for response when initializing therapy.

Max Dose: 20 mg PO daily.

FDA Approval: MDD (12 and up) and Generalized Anxiety Disorder (GAD).

Common Side Effects: Fatigue, GI upset, sexual dysfunction, insomnia, bruising, agitation, headache, nausea (better in 3–5 days).

Rare: *Seizures, hyponatremia, induction of mania, serotonin syndrome, bleeding, SIADH, and activation of suicidal ideation in those under 24.*

Monitoring: PHQ-9, ECG if QT prolongation. Height and weight on children.

Pearl: Lexapro has the best side effect profile of all SSRIs.

Contraindications: Taking MAO-I, pimozide, and known hypersensitivity to escitalopram. Avoid in untreated angle-closure glaucoma.

Black Box Warning: May increase suicidal thoughts in children, adolescents, and young adults (24 and younger).

Fluoxetine (Prozac)

Starting Dose: 20 mg PO daily. Can use 10 mg PO daily in elderly.

Titration: Increase by 20 mg PO daily after 1 week. Wait 4–6 weeks for response when initializing therapy.

Max Dose: 80 mg PO daily.

FDA Approval: MDD (8 and older), OCD (7 and older), PMDD, bulimia, panic disorder.

Common Side Effects: GI upset, sexual dysfunction, insomnia, anxiety, agitation, headache, dizziness, sweating, bruising, and nausea (better in 3–5 days).

Rare: *Seizures, hyponatremia, induction of mania, serotonin syndrome, bleeding, SIADH, and activation of suicidal ideation in those under 24.*

Monitoring: PHQ-9, ECG if QT prolongation. Height and weight on children.

Pearl: No need to taper off medication when discontinuing due to long half-life.

Contraindications: Taking MAO-I, thioridazine, pimozide, and known hypersensitivity to fluoxetine.

Black Box Warning: May increase suicidal thoughts in children, adolescents, and young adults (24 and younger).

Fluvoxamine CR (Luvox CR)

Starting Dose: 100 mg PO nightly.

Titration: Increase by 100 mg PO nightly every week.

Max Dose: 300 mg PO daily.

FDA Approval: Obsessive compulsive disorder and social anxiety disorder.

Common Side Effects: GI upset, sexual dysfunction, sweating, insomnia, agitation, headache, nausea better in 3–5 days.

Rare: *Seizures, hyponatremia, induction of mania, and activation of suicidal ideation in those under 24.*

Monitoring: None.

Pearl: Usually given at night due to sedation. Doses greater than 100 mg can be twice daily dosing to improve tolerability.

Contraindications: Taking MAO-I, thioridazine, pimozide, or tamoxifen.

Gabapentin (Neurontin)

Starting Dose: 100 mg PO BID.

Titration: Increase by 300–600 mg daily every 4–7 days.

Max Dose: Not much more benefit above 600 mg PO TID.

FDA Approval: Partial seizures, postherpetic neuralgia, restless leg syndrome (Extended release).

Off-Label Anxiety Disorders: Anxiety.

Common Side Effects: Sedation, dizziness, ataxia, peripheral edema, blurred vision, GI upset, heart burn, and dry mouth.

Rare: *Activation of suicidal ideation, anaphylaxis*, and *angioedema*.

Monitoring: GAD-7, monitor for sedation.

Pearl: Do not take antacid within 2 h of taking gabapentin. Taper over a minimum of 1 week.

Hydroxyzine (Vistaril)

Starting Dose: 25 mg PO every 6 h.

Titration: May go up in 25 mg increments q 6 h.

Max Dose: 100 mg four times daily.

FDA Approval: Anxiety and tension associated with psychoneurosis, pruritis due to allergic condition, histamine-mediated pruritis, premedication sedation, acute hysteria, anxiety withdrawal symptoms in alcoholics, nausea, and vomiting.

Off-Label: Insomnia.

Common Side Effects: Dry mouth, drowsiness, GI issues, headache, agitation.

Monitoring: GAD-7.

Pearl: Taken at first sign of anxiety.

Contraindication: Early stage pregnancy, patients with prolonged QT interval, and known hypersensitivity to hydroxyzine.

*****Beers List for drugs to avoid in the elderly*****

Mirtazapine (Remeron)—Noradrenergic and Specific Serotonergic Antidepressant (NaSSA)

Starting Dose: 15 mg PO nightly.

Titration: Increase by 15 mg per titration.

Max Dose: Typically, 45 mg PO nightly.

FDA Approval: Major Depressive Disorder (MDD).

Common Side Effects: Dry mouth, constipation, weight gain, sedation, dizziness, confusion, urinary retention, abnormal dreams, hypotension, QTc prolongation, and flu-like symptoms.

Rare: *Agranulocytosis, serotonin syndrome, hyponatremia, seizures, induction of mania, and activation of suicidal ideation in those under 24.*

Monitoring: PHQ-9. EKG may be prudent if taking other QTc prolonging drugs, especially in the geriatric population.

PEARL: More sedating at lower doses with 7.5 mg being most sedating. Often used for insomnia. Weight gain can be significant.

Contraindication: Patient taking an MAO-I.

Black Box Warning: May increase suicidal thoughts in children, adolescents, and young adults (24 and younger).

Paroxetine (Paxil)

Starting Dose:

Immediate Release: 20 mg PO daily. Can use 10 mg PO daily in elderly.

Controlled Release: 25 mg PO daily.

Titration:

Immediate Release: Increase by 10 mg PO daily, after 1 week. Wait 4–6 weeks for response when initializing therapy.

Controlled Release: 12.5 mg PO daily, after 1 week. Wait 4–6 weeks for response when initializing therapy.

Max Dose:

Immediate Release: 50 mg PO daily.

Controlled Release: 62.5 mg PO daily.

FDA Approval: MDD, OCD, panic disorder, SAD, PTSD, GAD, PMDD.

Common Side Effects: GI upset, sexual dysfunction, agitation, headache, sedation, dizziness, tremor, bruising, weight gain, nausea (better in 3–5 days).

Rare: *Seizures, hyponatremia, induction of mania, serotonin syndrome, bleeding, SIADH, and activation of suicidal ideation in those under 24.*

Monitoring: PHQ-9.

Pearl: May need to wean over several months for those who can't tolerate withdrawal effects.

Contraindications: Taking MAO-I, pimozide, and known hypersensitivity to Paroxetine.

Black Box Warning: May increase suicidal thoughts in children, adolescents, and young adults (24 and younger).

*****Beers List for drugs to avoid in the elderly*****

Pregabalin (Lyrica)

Starting Dose: 75 mg PO BID, 150 mg/day.

Titration: Increase by 150 mg/day weekly—BID or TID dosing.

Max Dose: 600 mg PO daily.

FDA Approval: Diabetic peripheral neuropathy, postherpetic neuralgia, neuropathic pain r/t spinal cord injury, and partial onset seizures.

Off-Label Anxiety Disorders: GAD, panic disorder, social anxiety disorder.

Common Side Effects: Sedation, dizziness, dry mouth, impaired attention, ataxia, fatigue, blurred vision, peripheral edema, diplopia, decreased libido, erectile dysfunction, tremor, irritability, GI upset, and weight gain.

Rare: *Activation of suicidal ideation.*

Monitoring: GAD-7.

Pearl: If given with additional sedating medication, titrate slowly after 1 week. Better tolerated with TID dosing.

Contraindication: Galactose intolerance, the Lapp lactase deficiency, or glucose-galactose malabsorption.

Sertraline (Zoloft)

Starting Dose: 50 mg PO daily. 25 mg PO daily in elderly.

Titration: Increase by 25–50 mg PO daily every week. Wait 4–6 weeks for response when initializing therapy.

Max Dose: 200 mg PO daily.

FDA Approval: Major Depressive Disorder (MDD), Obsessive Compulsive Disorder (OCD), Panic Disorder, Posttraumatic Stress Disorder (PTSD), Premenstrual Dysphoric Disorder (PMDD), social anxiety disorder.

Common Side Effects: GI upset, sexual dysfunction, agitation, headache, insomnia, sedation, sweating, bruising, and nausea (better in 3–5 days).

Rare: *Seizures, hyponatremia, induction of mania, hypotension, serotonin syndrome, bleeding, SIADH, and activation of suicidal ideation in those under 24.*

Monitoring: PHQ-9.

Contraindications: Taking MAO-I, pimozide, and known hypersensitivity to Sertraline. Avoid in untreated Angle-Closure Glaucoma.

Black Box Warning: May increase suicidal thoughts in children, adolescents, and young adults (24 and younger).

Trazodone (Desyrel)—Serotonin 2 Antagonist/Reuptake Inhibitor (SARI)

Starting Dose: 150 mg in divided doses.

Titration: Increase by 50 mg PO nightly.

Max Dose: 400 mg PO daily.

FDA Approval: Major Depressive Disorder (MDD).

Common Side Effects: GI upset, sexual dysfunction, insomnia, agitation, sedation, dizziness, blurred vision, urinary retention, headache, nausea better in 3–5 days.

Rare: *Seizures, QTC prolongation, serotonin syndrome, hyponatremia, abnormal bleeding, orthostatic hypotension/syncope, hyponatremia, priapism, induction of mania, and activation of suicidal ideation in those under 24.*

Monitoring: PHQ-9. EKG may be prudent if taking other QTc prolonging drugs, especially in the geriatric population.

PEARL: Often used for insomnia due to sedating properties at lower doses.

Contraindication: Patient taking an MAO-I.

Black Box Warning: May increase suicidal thoughts in children, adolescents, and young adults (24 and younger).

Venlafaxine XR (Effexor XR)

Starting Dose: 37.5 mg PO daily.

Titration: Increase by 37.5 mg PO daily in 1 week. Then may titrate by 75 mg PO daily. Wait 4–6 weeks (on 75 mg dose) for response when initializing therapy.

Max Dose: 375 mg PO daily.

FDA Approval: Depression, GAD, SAD, panic disorder, separation anxiety disorder.

Common Side Effects: Increased blood pressure, GI upset, sexual dysfunction, insomnia, agitation, anxiety, sweating, abnormal vision, headache, nausea (better in 3–5 days).

Rare: *Seizures, hyponatremia, induction of mania, serotonin syndrome, SIADH, and activation of suicidal ideation in those under 24.*

Monitoring: PHQ-9 and blood pressure at each visit.

Pearls: Higher doses are associated with more side effects. Immediate release forms available but are more prone to discontinuation syndrome. Effexor can be difficult to wean; alternative strategies may need to be used and length of titration may take months. Patients commonly report "brain zaps" while discontinuing or even missing a dose. Medication is renally cleared and may need dose reduction of 25–50% in renal disease.

Contraindications: Uncontrolled angle-closure glaucoma or taking an MAO-I.

Black Box Warning: May increase suicidal thoughts in children, adolescents, and young adults (24 and younger).

Vilazodone (Viibryd)—SSRI Plus 5HT1A Partial Agonist

Starting Dose: 10 mg PO daily.

Titration: Increase by 10 mg PO daily every week. Wait 4–6 weeks for response when initializing therapy.

Max Dose: 40 mg PO daily.

FDA Approval: Major Depressive Disorder (MDD).

Common Side Effects: GI upset, sexual dysfunction, dry mouth, bruising, insomnia, dizziness, agitation, headache, and nausea (better in 3–5 days).

Rare: *Seizures, hyponatremia, induction of mania, serotonin syndrome, bleeding, SIADH, and activation of suicidal ideation in those under 24.*

Monitoring: PHQ-9.

Pearl: Should be taken with food to aid in absorption.

Contraindications: Taking MAO-I. Avoid in untreated angle-closure glaucoma.

Black Box Warning: May increase suicidal thoughts in children, adolescents, and young adults (24 and younger).

Vortioxetine (Trintellix)—SSRI Plus 5H1 Receptor Modulator

Starting Dose: 10 mg PO daily. 5 mg PO daily in elderly.

Titration: Increase by 10 mg every week. Wait 4–6 weeks for response when initializing therapy.

Max Dose: 20 mg PO daily.

FDA Approval: Major Depressive Disorder (MDD).

Common Side Effects: GI upset, sexual dysfunction, and constipation.

Rare: *Seizures, hyponatremia, induction of mania, serotonin syndrome, and activation of suicidal ideation in those under 24.*

Monitoring: PHQ-9.

Contraindications: Taking MAO-I. Avoid in untreated angle-closure glaucoma.

Black Box Warning: May increase suicidal thoughts in children, adolescents, and young adults (24 and younger).

Benzodiazepines

Benzodiazepines are on the Beers List for drugs to avoid in the elderly

Alprazolam (Xanax)

Starting Dose: 0.25 mg PO (Daily to TID) PRN.
Titration: 0.25–0.5 mg PO (Daily to TID).
Max Dose: 3 mg/day.
FDA Approval: Generalized anxiety disorder and panic disorder.
Off-Label Disorders: Other anxiety disorders, anxiety associated with depression, IBS, acute mania, acute psychosis, and catatonia.
Common Side Effects: Sedation, fatigue, depression, dizziness, ataxia, slurred speech, weakness, forgetfulness, confusion, hyperexcitability, nervousness, dry mouth, mania, hypotension, respiratory depression.
Rare: *Hepatic dysfunction, renal dysfunction, blood dyscrasias.*
Monitoring: GAD-7.
Pearl: Withdrawal can occur with prolonged use, will need expert guidance on discontinuing medication. Do not mix with alcohol.
Contraindicated: Angle-closure glaucoma or with concomitant azole use.

Clonazepam (Klonopin)

Starting Dose: 0.25 mg PO (Daily to BID) PRN.
Titration: 0.25–0.5 mg PO (Daily) PRN.
Max Dose: 4 mg/day.
FDA Approval: Panic disorder, Lennox-Gastaut syndrome, akinetic seizure, myoclonic seizure, and absence seizure.

Off-Label Disorders: Atonic seizures, other anxiety disorders, insomnia, and catatonia.

Common Side Effects: Sedation, fatigue, depression, dizziness, ataxia, slurred speech, weakness, forgetfulness, confusion, hyperexcitability, nervousness, dry mouth, mania, hypotension, respiratory depression.

Rare: *Hepatic dysfunction, renal dysfunction, blood dyscrasias.*

Pearl: Withdrawal can occur with prolonged use, will need expert guidance on discontinuing medication. Do not mix with alcohol.

Contraindicated: Angle-closure glaucoma or with concomitant azole use.

Clorazepate (Tranxene)

Starting Dose: 7.5 mg PO BID – 15 mg/day.

Titration: 7.5 mg PO TID.

Max Dose: 90 mg/day.

FDA Approval: Anxiety disorder, symptoms of anxiety, acute alcohol withdrawal.

Off-Label Disorders: Partial seizures and catatonia.

Common Side Effects: Sedation, fatigue, depression, dizziness, ataxia, slurred speech, weakness, forgetfulness, confusion, hyperexcitability, nervousness, dry mouth, mania, hypotension, and respiratory depression.

Rare: *Hepatic dysfunction, renal dysfunction, blood dyscrasias.*

Monitoring: GAD-7.

Pearl: Withdrawal can occur with prolonged use, will need expert guidance on discontinuing medication.

Contraindicated in angle-closure glaucoma.

Lorazepam (Ativan)

Starting Dose: 2 mg/day broken down into TID dosing.

Titration: 0.5 mg PO TID or 1.5 mg daily.

Max Dose: 10 mg/day.

FDA Approval: Anxiety disorder, anxiety associated with depressive symptoms, status epilepticus, preanesthetic.

Off-Label Disorders: Insomnia, alcohol withdrawal psychosis, panic disorder, acute mania, acute psychosis, catatonia.

Common Side Effects: Sedation, fatigue, depression, dizziness, ataxia, slurred speech, weakness, forgetfulness, confusion, hyperexcitability, nervousness, dry mouth, mania, hypotension, respiratory depression.

Rare: *Hepatic dysfunction, renal dysfunction, blood dyscrasias.*

Monitoring: GAD-7.

Pearl: Withdrawal can occur with prolonged use, will need expert guidance on discontinuing medication.

Contraindicated: Angle-closure glaucoma or with concomitant azole use.

Oxazepam (Serax)

Starting Dose: Mild to moderate: 10–15 mg PO TID/QID. Range: 30–60 mg/day.

Severe: Up to 30 mg PO TID/QID. Range: 45–120 mg/day.

Titration: Titration usually not necessary.

Max Dose: 120 mg/day.

FDA Approval: Anxiety, anxiety associated with depression, and alcohol withdrawal.

Off-Label Disorders: Catatonia.

Common Side Effects: Sedation, fatigue, depression, dizziness, ataxia, slurred speech, weakness, forgetfulness, confusion, hyperexcitability, nervousness, dry mouth, mania, hypotension, respiratory depression.

Rare: *Hepatic dysfunction, renal dysfunction, blood dyscrasias.*

Monitoring: GAD-7.

Pearl: Withdrawal can occur with prolonged use, will need expert guidance on discontinuing medication.

Contraindicated: Angle-closure glaucoma or with concomitant azole use.

Temazepam (Restoril)

Starting Dose: 15 mg PO nightly.

Titration: 15 mg if tolerated but ineffective.

Max Dose: 30 mg PO nightly.

FDA Approval: Short-term treatment of insomnia (7–10 days).

Common Side Effects: Sedation, fatigue, depression, dizziness, ataxia, slurred speech, weakness, forgetfulness, confusion, hyperexcitability, nervousness, hypersalivation, dry mouth, rebound insomnia.

Rare: *Respiratory depression, hallucinations, mania, hypotension, hepatic dysfunction, renal dysfunction, and blood dyscrasias.*

Monitoring: None.

Contraindications: Pregnancy, angle-closure glaucoma, allergy.

Pearl: Usually not written for more than a 1 month supply. Do not mix with alcohol or opioids.

Insomnia Medications

Daridorexant (QUVIVIQ)—Dual Orexin Receptor Antagonist/Hypnotic

Starting Dose: 25 mg PO nightly.

Titration: 25 mg PO nightly after 7 days.

Max Dose: 50 mg per night.

FDA Approval: Insomnia (sleep maintenance and sleep onset).

Common Side Effects: Sedation, headache.

Uncommon/Rare: *Sleep paralysis, hypnagogic/hypnopompic hallucinations, symptoms similar to mild cataplexy.*

Monitoring: None.

Contraindications: Narcolepsy, not recommended in someone taking strong CYP450 3A4 inhibitor.

Pearl: Not restricted to short-term use. Do not use unless there is 7 h before needing to wake. Maximum dose is 25 mg in those taking mild CYP450 3A4 inhibitors.

Doxepin (Silenor)

Starting Dose: 3 mg PO nightly.

Titration: Increase by 3 mg PO nightly.

Max Dose: 6 mg typical for insomnia. Max dose is 300 mg/day.

FDA Approval: Sleep maintenance insomnia, depression, and anxiety associated with alcoholism and organic disease, psychotic depressive disorders with associated anxiety, involutional depression, manic-depressive disorder, and psychoneurotic patient with depression and/or anxiety.

Common Side Effects: Sedation, increased appetite, nausea, diarrhea, heartburn, fatigue, weakness, headache, anxiety, sexual dysfunction, weight gain.

Uncommon: *Paralytic ileus, hyperthermia, lowered seizure threshold, orthostatic hypotension, arrhythmias, QTc prolongation, hepatic failure, rare induction of mania.*

Monitoring: EKG prior to administering if over 50, taking QTc prolonging drugs, or certain cardiac conditions. Weight before initiating and following BMI every 3 months.

Contraindications: History of QTc prolongation, recent myocardial infarction, uncompensated heart failure, angle-closure glaucoma, severe urinary retention, taking drugs that inhibit TCA metabolism.

Black Box Warning: May increase suicidal thoughts in children, adolescents, and young adults (24 and younger).

*****Beers List for drugs to avoid (> 6 mg) in the elderly*****

Eszopiclone (Lunesta)

Starting Dose: 1 mg PO nightly.

Titration: 1 mg PO nightly every week.

Max Dose: 3 mg PO nightly.

FDA Approval: Insomnia.

Common Side Effects: Unpleasant taste, sedation, headache, dizziness, dry mouth, dose-dependent amnesia,

Uncommon: *Respiratory depression, angioedema.*

Monitoring: None.

Contraindications: Pt has experienced episode of complex sleep behaviors while taking a sleep medication.

*****Beers List for drugs to avoid >90 days in the elderly*****

Lemborexant (Dayvigo)—Dual Orexin Receptor Antagonist/Hypnotic

Starting Dose: 5 mg PO nightly.

Titration: 5 mg PO nightly after 7 days.

Max Dose: 10 mg per night.

FDA Approval: Insomnia (sleep maintenance and sleep onset).

Common Side Effects: Sedation, headache, dizziness, abnormal dreams, sleep paralysis, hypnagogic/hypnopompic hallucinations.

Rare: Sleep paralysis, hypnagogic/hypnopompic hallucinations, symptoms similar to mild cataplexy.

Monitoring: None.

Contraindications: Narcolepsy, not recommended in someone taking strong CYP450 3A4 inhibitor.

PEARL: Not restricted to short-term use. Do not use unless there is 7 h before needing to wake. Maximum dose is 5 mg in those taking mild CYP450 3A4 inhibitors.

Ramelteon (Rozerem)—Melatonin 1 and 2 Receptor Agonist

Starting Dose: 8 mg PO nightly.

Titration: None.

Max Dose: 8 mg.

FDA Approval: Sleep onset insomnia.

Common Side Effects: Sedation, dizziness, fatigue, headache, respiratory depression, angioedema.

Rare: *Angioedema, respiratory depression when taken with other CNS depressants in overdose.*

Monitoring: None.

Contraindications: Hepatic impairment.

Pearl: May titrate up by 8 mg prior to calling medication trial a failure. Only approved for 8 mg per night.

Suvorexant (Belsomra)—Dual Orexin Receptor Antagonist/Hypnotic

Starting Dose: 10 mg PO nightly.

Titration: 5 mg PO nightly after 7 days.

Max Dose: 20 mg per night.

FDA Approval: Insomnia (sleep maintenance and sleep onset).

Common Side Effects: Sedation, headache, abnormal dreams.

Rare: *Sleep paralysis, hypnagogic/hypnopompic hallucinations, symptoms similar to mild cataplexy.*

Monitoring: None.

Contraindications: Narcolepsy, not recommended in someone taking strong or moderate CYP450 3A4 inhibitor.

Pearl: Not restricted to short-term use. Do not use unless there is 7 h before needing to wake.

Temazepam (Restoril)

Starting Dose: 15 mg PO nightly.

Titration: 15 mg if tolerated but ineffective.

Max Dose: 30 mg PO nightly.

FDA Approval: Short-term treatment of insomnia (7–10 days).

Common Side Effects: Sedation, fatigue, depression, dizziness, ataxia, slurred speech, weakness, forgetfulness, confusion, hyperexcitability, nervousness, hypersalivation, dry mouth, rebound insomnia.

Rare: *Respiratory depression, hallucinations, mania, hypotension, hepatic dysfunction, renal dysfunction, and blood dyscrasias.*

Monitoring: None.

Contraindications: Pregnancy, angle-closure glaucoma, allergy.

Pearl: Usually not written for more than a 1 month supply. Do not mix with alcohol or opioids.

*****Beers List for drugs to avoid >90 days in the elderly*****

Zaleplon (Sonata)

Starting Dose: 10 mg PO nightly.

Titration: May increase to 20 mg PO nightly.

Max Dose: 20 mg PO nightly.

FDA Approval: Short-term treatment of insomnia.

Common Side Effects: Sedation, headache, dizziness, ataxia, dose-dependent amnesia, respiratory depression, angioedema.

Rare: *Respiratory depression when taken with other CNS depressants in overdose, angioedema.*

Monitoring: None.

Contraindications: Pt has experienced episode of complex sleep behaviors while taking a sleep.

Pearl: Pt with lower bodyweight may only require 5 mg nightly.

*****Beers List for drugs to avoid >90 days in the elderly*****

Zolpidem (Ambien)

Starting Dose: 10 mg PO nightly for men/5 mg PO nightly for women.

Titration: N/A.

Max Dose: 10 mg PO nightly.

FDA Approval: Short-term treatment of insomnia (7–10 days).

Common Side Effects: Sedation, headache, dizziness, dry mouth, dose-dependent amnesia.

Rare: *Respiratory depression* especially when taken with other CNS depressants in overdose, *angioedema*, and hallucinations.

Monitoring: None.

Contraindications: Pt has experienced episode of complex sleep behaviors while taking a sleep medication.

*****Beers List for drugs to avoid >90 days in the elderly*****

Zolpidem (Ambien CR)

Starting Dose: 12.5 mg PO nightly for men/6.25 mg PO nightly for women.
Titration: N/A.
Max Dose: 12.5 mg PO nightly.
FDA Approval: Short-term treatment of insomnia (7–10 days).
Common Side Effects: Sedation, headache, dizziness, dry mouth, dose-dependent amnesia.
Rare: *Respiratory depression* especially when taken with other CNS depressants in overdose, *angioedema*, and hallucinations.
Monitoring: None.
Contraindications: Pt has experienced episode of complex sleep behaviors while taking a sleep medication.

*****Beers List for drugs to avoid >90 days in the elderly*****

Zolpidem (Intermezzo)

Starting Dose: 3.5 mg sublingual nightly in men, 1.75 mg sublingual nightly in women and elderly.
Titration: N/A.
Max Dose: 10 mg sublingual nightly.
FDA Approval: Short-term treatment of insomnia (7–10 days).
Common Side Effects: Sedation, headache, dizziness, dry mouth, dose-dependent amnesia.
Rare: *Respiratory depression* especially when taken with other CNS depressants in overdose, *angioedema*, and hallucinations.
Monitoring: None.
Contraindications: Pt has experienced episode of complex sleep behaviors while taking a sleep medication.
Pearl: Taken in the middle of the night if 4 h of bedtime remain.

*****Beers List for drugs to avoid >90 days in the elderly*****

Mood Stabilizers

Carbamazepine (Equetro)

Starting Dose: 200 mg PO twice daily.

Titration: Increase by 200 mg PO daily every week.

Max Dose: 1200 mg/day.

FDA Approval: Acute mania (bipolar), mixed mania (bipolar), partial seizures with complex symptomology, generalized tonic-clonic seizures, mixed seizure patterns, trigeminal neuralgia pain.

Common Side Effects: Rash, benign leukopenia, GI upset, dry mouth, blurred vision, sedation, dizziness, unsteadiness, and confusion.

Rare: *Aplastic anemia, agranulocytosis, severe dermatologic reactions such as SJS and purpura, anaphylaxis, induction of psychosis or mania, SIADH, and activation of suicidal ideation and behavior.*

Monitoring: Initiation: CBC, CMP, and thyroid. During treatment: CBC q 2–4 weeks for 2 months and then q 3–6 months. CMP and thyroid q 6–12 months.

Contraindications: History of bone marrow suppression, allergy to carbamazepine, proven allergy to any tricyclic compound, and positive test for HLA-B*1502 allele.

Black Box Warning: Serious dermatologic reactions (toxic epidermal necrolysis and Stevens-Johnson syndrome) and aplastic anemia/agranulocytosis.

Divalproex (Depakote ER)

Starting Dose: Mania: 25 mg/kg/day.

Titration: 10–20 mg/kg/day.

Max Dose: 60 mg/kg/day.

FDA Approval: Acute mania and mixed episodes, seizures, migraine prophylaxis, bipolar maintenance.

Common Side Effects: Sedation, tremor, dizziness, abdominal pain, N/V/D, reduced appetite, constipation, heart burn, weight gain, ataxia, asthenia, headache, *tachycardia/bradycardia.*

Rare: *Hepatotoxicity, pancreatitis, DRESS, activation of suicidal ideation.*

Monitoring: CBC, CMP at baseline. LFT frequently. If tired or confused, draw ammonia.

Contraindications: Pancreatitis, severe liver disease, urea cycle disorder.

Pearls: Don't use with women with PCOS. Only use half dose if adding Lamictal (Blue starter pack).

Black Box Warning: Increased risk of pancreatitis and liver failure.

Lamotrigine (Lamictal) (Goal is 150–250 mg)

Starting Dose: 25 mg PO daily.

Titration: Increase by 25 mg every 2 weeks.

Max Dose: 400 mg PO daily and higher have been used.

FDA Approval: Maintenance treatment of bipolar 1, partial seizures, and tonic/clonic seizures.

Common Side Effects: Benign rash, blurred vision, dizziness, ataxia, sedation, headache, tremor, insomnia, poor coordination, and fatigue.

Rare: *Serious rash, Stevens-Johnson syndrome, blood dyscrasias, aseptic meningitis, hemophagocytic lymphohistiocytosis.*

Monitoring: Creatinine at baseline. Eye exam for prolonged treatment. Assess for depression and SI.

Pearls: If adding Depakote, only use half the dose instead of full Depakote dose. Start 125 mg PO QHS. With slow titration, may need atypical such as Vraylar. Can take months for proper titration.

Black Box Warning: Life-threatening serious rashes including Stevens-Johnson syndrome, toxic epidermal necrolysis, and/or rash-related death.

Lithium (Best for Mania and Depression. As Well as Suicidality. Helps Preserve Brain Size)

Starting Dose: 300 mg PO TID.

Titration: Increase by 300 mg/day every 3 days.

Max Dose: 1800 mg PO daily.

FDA Approval: Manic episodes, acute mania/mixed mania, maintenance treatment for manic-depressive patients with history of mania, and bipolar maintenance.

Common Side Effects: Ataxia, dysarthria, delirium, tremor, memory problems, polyura, polydipsia, diarrhea, nausea, weight gain, goiter, hypothyroidism, acne, rash, alopecia, metallic taste, leukocytosis, renal impairment, nephrogenic diabetes insipidus, arrhythmia, sick sinus syndrome, hypotension.

Monitoring: CBC, CMP, TSH baseline, 1 month after treatment and then q 6 months. Drug levels twice weekly until stable then q 2 months until chronic steady dose. Parathyroid for low calcium. Lithium level goals: Acute treatment: 1.0–1.5 mEq/L, Chronic treatment: 0.6–1.2 mEq/L.

Pearls: Decreased risk of suicidality.

Contraindications: Severe kidney disease, severe cardiovascular disease, Brugada syndrome, severe dehydration, or sodium depletion.

Black Box Warning: Lithium toxicity is closely related to lithium blood levels and can occur at doses close to therapeutic levels.

Non-stimulant ADHD Medications

Atomoxetine (Strattera)

Starting Dose: 40 mg PO daily.

Titration: Increase to 80 mg after 7 days and then to 100 mg PO daily in 2–4 weeks.

Max Dose: 100 mg/day.

FDA Approval: ADHD in children ages 6 and older.

Common Side Effects: Sedation, fatigue, decreased appetite, increased heart rate and blood pressure, insomnia, dizziness, irritability, dry mouth, constipation, nausea, vomiting, abdominal pain, heart burn, sexual dysfunction, anxiety, agitation, and aggression.

Rare: *Cardiovascular adverse effects, severe liver damage, hypomania, priapism, activation of suicidal ideation.*

Monitoring: Blood pressure at initiation, after dose increase, and periodically.

Contraindications: Taking an MAO-I, history of pheochromocytoma, severe cardiovascular disorder, angle-closure glaucoma.

Black Box Warning: Risk of suicidality in children/adolescents with ADHD, especially within first month of treatment.

Clonidine (Kapvay)—Ages 6–17

Starting Dose: Extended Release 0.1 mg PO nightly.

Titration: Extended Release: 0.1 mg per week, after 3–4 weeks.

Max Dose: Extended Release: 4 mg.

FDA Approval: Hypertension, ADHD in children 6–17 years old.

Common Side Effects: Sedation, dizziness, abdominal pain, nausea, fatigue, weakness, hypotension, dry mouth, constipation, and bradycardia.

Rare: *Sinus bradycardia, atrioventricular block, hypertensive encephalopathy*, *CVA*, and *death* (during withdrawal).

Monitoring: Blood pressure regularly.

*****Beers List for drugs to avoid in the elderly*****

Guanfacine (Intuniv) Ages 6–17

Starting Dose: Extended Release: 1 mg PO daily.

Titration: Extended Release: Increase by 1 mg PO daily every week.

Max Dose: 4 mg/day.

FDA Approval: Hypertension, ADHD in children 6–17 years old.

Common Side Effects: Dry mouth, constipation, hypotension, insomnia, agitation, dizziness, lightheadedness, headache, fatigue, blurred vision, nausea, orthostatic hypotension, *sinus bradycardia*.

Monitoring: None.

Pearl: Given during the day for hyperarousal, not typically given to treat nightmares.

*****Beers List for drugs to avoid in the elderly*****

Viloxazine (Qelbree) (12 Years Old +)

Starting Dose: 200 mg PO daily.

Titration: Increase 200 mg PO daily each week.

Max Dose: 600 mg/day, Ages 12–17: 400 mg/day.

FDA Approval: ADHD ages 6 and up.

Common Side Effects: Fatigue, sleepiness, insomnia, irritability, headache, decreased appetite, nausea, vomiting, dry mouth, constipation, increased heart rate and blood pressure.

Rare: *Hypomania.*

Monitoring: Blood pressure at initiation, after dose increase, and periodically throughout treatment.

Contraindications: Taking MAO-I inhibitor, history of pheochromocytoma, angle-closure glaucoma, and severe cardiovascular disorder.

Pearl: If too sedating, take at night to reduce daytime drowsiness.

Black Box Warning: Risk of suicidality in children/adolescents with ADHD, especially within first month of treatment.

PTSD Medications

Clonidine (Catapres)

Starting Dose: 0.1 mg PO daily.

Titration: Increase by 0.1 mg PO daily every week.

Max Dose: 0.4 mg/day.

FDA Approval: Hypertension, ADHD in children 6–17 years old.

Common Side Effects: Sedation, dizziness, abdominal pain, nausea, fatigue, weakness, hypotension, dry mouth, constipation, and bradycardia.

Rare: *Sinus bradycardia, atrioventricular block, hypertensive encephalopathy, CVA*, and *death* (during withdrawal).

Monitoring: Blood pressure regularly.

*****Beers List for drugs to avoid in the elderly*****

Prazosin (Minipress)

Starting Dose: 1 mg PO nightly.

Titration: Increase by 1–2 mg PO nightly every couple weeks.

Max Dose: 40 mg/day.

FDA Approval: Hypertension.

Common Side Effects: Dizziness, lightheadedness, headache, fatigue, blurred vision, nausea, orthostatic hypotension, *syncope with sudden loss of consciousness.*

Rare: *Priapism.*

Monitoring: None.

Pearl: Given at night to treat nightmares. May also be given during the day to help combat hyperarousal.

*****Beers List for drugs to avoid in the elderly*****

Second-Generation Antipsychotics

"Beer's List for off-label use. Should only be used when FDA indicated and at lowest effective dose."

Aripiprazole (Abilify)

Starting Dose: 2–5 mg PO daily.
Titration: Increase by 2–5 mg PO daily every week.
Max Dose: 15 mg PO daily.
FDA Approval: Depression adjunct, schizophrenia, bipolar maintenance, autism-related irritability, Tourette's disorder in children ages 6–18, and agitation associated with schizophrenia or bipolar disorder (IM Abilify).
Common Side Effects: Dizziness, insomnia, akathisia, activation, nausea, vomiting, constipation, headache, orthostatic hypotension, tardive dyskinesia.
Rare: *Impulse control problems (gambling), hyperglycemia, neuroleptic malignant syndrome (NMS), seizures.*
Monitoring: PHQ-9, BMI every 3 months, lipid panel, and A1c annually. Waist circumference, blood pressure, fasting plasma glucose, and fasting lipid profile prior to start, within 3 months and then annually. AIMS score every 3–6 months.
Pearl: Injectable form available.
Black Box Warning: Elderly dementia patients who take Abilify have a higher risk of death. May increase suicidal thoughts in children, adolescents, and young adults.

Asenapine (Saphris)

Starting Dose: Mania: 10 mg sublingual BID (20 mg/day).
Titration: May reduce to 5 mg sublingual BID (10 mg/day) if adverse effects.
Max Dose: 20 mg/day.
FDA Approval: Schizophrenia, mania/mixed mania, and bipolar maintenance.
Common Side Effects: Increased risk for diabetes and dyslipidemia, dizziness, sedation, dry mouth, constipation, weight gain, edema, musculoskeletal pain, orthostatic hypotension, tardive dyskinesia.
Rare: *Type-1 hypersensitivity reactions, hyperglycemia (ketoacidosis), NMS.*

Monitoring: PHQ-9, BMI every 3 months, lipid panel, and A1c annually. Waist circumference, blood pressure, fasting plasma glucose, and fasting lipid profile prior to start, within 3 months and then annually. AIMS score every 3–6 months.

Black Box Warning: Elderly dementia patients who take Saphris have a higher risk of death. May increase suicidal thoughts in children, adolescents, and young adults (24 and younger).

Brexpiprazole (Rexulti)

Starting Dose: 0.5–1 mg once daily.

Titration: May increase by 1 mg daily every week.

Max Dose: 3 mg PO daily.

FDA Approval: Treatment resistant depression used as adjunct and schizophrenia.

Common Side Effects: Akathisia, weight gain, sedation, headache, and tardive dyskinesia.

Rare: *Impulse control problems (gambling), hyperglycemia, neuroleptic malignant syndrome, seizures.*

Monitoring: PHQ-9, BMI every 3 months, lipid panel, and A1c annually. Waist circumference, blood pressure, fasting plasma glucose, and fasting lipid profile prior to start, within 3 months and then annually. AIMS score every 3–6 months.

Black Box Warning: Elderly dementia patients who take Rexulti have a higher risk of death. May increase suicidal thoughts in children, adolescents, and young adults (24 and younger).

Cariprazine (Vraylar)

Starting Dose: 1.5 mg PO daily.

Titration: Up to 3 mg after 14 days.

Max Dose: 3 mg.

FDA Approval: Schizophrenia acute and maintenance, acute mania/mixed mood, bipolar 1 (depression). MDD adjunct.

Common Side Effects: Akathisia, EPS, restlessness, GI distress, sedation, tardive dyskinesia.

Rare: *Hyperglycemia, neuroleptic malignant syndrome, and seizures.*

Monitoring: BMI monthly × 3 months then every 3 months. Blood pressure, fasting plasma glucose, fasting lipid panel within

3 months and then annually. More often if at risk for metabolic syndrome.

Pearl: Side effects may develop weeks later due to long half-life. 1.5 mg dose typically more effective for depressive symptoms.

Black Box Warning: Elderly dementia patients who take Vraylar have a higher risk of death. May increase suicidal thoughts in children, adolescents, and young adults.

Lumateperone (Caplyta)

Starting Dose: 42 mg.

Titration: None needed.

Max 42 mg.

FDA Approval: Schizophrenia, bipolar depression.

Common Side Effects: Sedation, nausea, dry mouth, tardive dyskinesia.

Uncommon: *Hyperglycemia, neuroleptic malignant syndrome, stroke, orthostatic hypotension, low white blood cell count,* and *seizures*.

Monitoring: BMI monthly × 3 months then every 3 months. Blood pressure, fasting plasma glucose, fasting lipid panel within 3 months and then monthly. More often if at risk for metabolic syndrome. AIMS score every 3–6 months.

Caveats: Not known for metabolic side effects. New dosage forms available: 10 mg, 21 mg, and 42 mg.

Black Box Warning: Elderly dementia patients who take Abilify have a higher risk of death. May increase suicidal thoughts in children, adolescents, and young adults.

Lurasidone (Latuda)

Starting Dose: 20 mg PO daily with largest meal.

Titration: Increase by 5–10 mg PO daily every week.

Max Dose: 120 mg PO daily.

FDA Approval: Schizophrenia, bipolar depression.

Common Side Effects: Sedation, akathisia, nausea, hyperprolactinemia, increased risk of diabetes and dyslipidemia, tardive dyskinesia.

Rare: *Tachycardia/first-degree AV block, hyperglycemia (ketoacidosis), NMS, seizures.*

Monitoring: BMI monthly × 3 months then every 3 months. Blood pressure, fasting plasma glucose, fasting lipid panel within 3 months and then monthly. More often if at risk for metabolic syndrome. AIMS score every 3–6 months.

Caveats: Give with >350 calories. Used in depressed state, watch for s/s of mania.

Contraindications: Taking a strong CYP 3A4 inhibitor/inducer (ketoconazole, rifampin), history of angioedema.

Black Box Warning: Elderly dementia patients who take Abilify have a higher risk of death. May increase suicidal thoughts in children, adolescents, and young adults.

Olanzapine (Zyprexa)

Starting Dose: 5 mg to 10 mg PO nightly.

Titration: 5 mg PO nightly every week.

Max Dose: 20 mg/day.

FDA Approval: Treatment-resistant depression, schizophrenia, bipolar maintenance, bipolar depression.

Common Side Effects: Increased risk for diabetes and dyslipidemia, dizziness, sedation, dry mouth, constipation, weight gain, edema, musculoskeletal pain, orthostatic hypotension, tardive dyskinesia.

Rare: *DRESS, hyperglycemia (ketoacidosis), NMS, seizures.*

Monitoring: GAD-7, BMI every 3 months, lipid panel, and A1c annually. Waist circumference, blood pressure, fasting plasma glucose, and fasting lipid profile prior to start, within 3 months and then annually. AIMS score every 3–6 months.

Contraindications: Risk of angle-closure glaucoma, unstable cardiac condition.

Black Box Warning: Elderly dementia patients who take Zyprexa have a higher risk of death. May increase suicidal thoughts in children, adolescents, and young adults (24 and younger).

Olanzapine-Fluoxetine (Symbyax)

Starting Dose: 6 mg/25 mg mg PO daily.

Titration: Increase by 3 mg of olanzapine or 25 mg of fluoxetine.

Max Dose: 18 mg/75 mg mg PO daily.

FDA Approval: Treatment-resistant depression, schizophrenia, bipolar maintenance, bipolar depression.

Common Side Effects: Increased risk of diabetes and dyslipidemia, dizziness, sedation, dry mouth, constipation, weight gain, edema, tachycardia, musculoskeletal pain, orthostatic hypotension, tardive dyskinesia.

Rare: *DRESS, hyperglycemia, neuroleptic malignant syndrome, and seizures.*

Monitoring: PHQ-9, BMI every 3 months, lipid panel, and A1c annually. Waist circumference, blood pressure, fasting plasma glucose, and fasting lipid profile prior to start, within 3 months and then annually. AIMS score every 3–6 months.

Contraindications: Known risk of angle-closure glaucoma or unstable cardiac condition.

Black Box Warning: Elderly dementia patients who take Symbyax have a higher risk of death. May increase suicidal thoughts in children, adolescents, and young adults (24 and younger).

Quetiapine (Seroquel)

Starting Dose: 50 mg PO BID.

Titration: 100 mg/day. Once at 400 mg/day, may increase by 200 mg/day.

Max Dose: 800 mg PO daily.

FDA Approval: MDD, bipolar depression, bipolar maintenance, schizophrenia.

Common Side Effects: GI upset, sexual dysfunction, insomnia, agitation, sedation, dizziness, urinary retention, headache, weight loss, myalgia, sweating, anorexia, hypertension, and nausea better in 3–5 days.

Rare: *Neuroleptic malignant syndrome, hyperglycemia, and seizures.*

Monitoring: PHQ-9, BMI every 3 months, lipid panel, and A1c annually. Waist circumference, blood pressure, fasting plasma glucose, and fasting lipid profile prior to start, within 3 months and then annually. AIMS score every 3–6 months.

Pearl: Known for sedating properties, could be useful insomnia adjunct in doses up to 100 mg.

Black Box Warning: Elderly dementia patients who take Seroquel have a higher risk of death. May increase suicidal thoughts in children, adolescents, and young adults (24 and younger).

Quetiapine XR (Seroquel XR)

Starting Dose: 50 mg PO nightly.

Titration: Increase by 50–100 mg PO nightly every week.

Max Dose: Usually 300 mg PO daily for depression.

FDA Approval: MDD, bipolar depression, bipolar maintenance, schizophrenia.

Common Side Effects: GI upset, sexual dysfunction, insomnia, agitation, sedation, dizziness, urinary retention, headache, weight loss, myalgia, sweating, anorexia, hypertension, and nausea better in 3–5 days.

Rare: *Agranulocytosis, leukopenia, neutropenia, neuroleptic malignant syndrome, and seizures.*

Monitoring: PHQ-9, BMI every 3 months, lipid panel, and A1c annually. Waist circumference, blood pressure, fasting plasma glucose, and fasting lipid profile prior to start, within 3 months and then annually. AIMS score every 3–6 months.

Pearl: Known for sedating properties, could be useful insomnia adjunct.

Black Box Warning: Elderly dementia patients who take Seroquel have a higher risk of death. May increase suicidal thoughts in children, adolescents, and young adults (24 and younger).

Risperidone (Risperdal)

Starting Dose: 0.5 mg PO BID (1 mg/day).

Titration: Increase by 1 mg/day, every day.

Max Dose: 16 mg/day.

FDA Approval: Schizophrenia, acute mania/mixed mania, autism-related irritability in children, and bipolar maintenance.

Common Side Effects: Increased risk for diabetes and dyslipidemia, drug-induced parkinsonism, hyperprolactinemia, dizziness, insomnia, anxiety, sedation, GI distress, weight gain, sexual dysfunction, tardive dyskinesia, and orthostatic hypotension.

Uncommon/Rare: *Hyperglycemia, neuroleptic malignant syndrome, seizures.*

Monitoring: PHQ-9, BMI every 3 months, lipid panel, and A1c annually. Waist circumference, blood pressure, fasting plasma glucose, and fasting lipid profile prior to start, within 3 months and then annually. AIMS score every 3–6 months.

Black Box Warning: Elderly dementia patients who take Zyprexa have a higher risk of death. May increase suicidal thoughts in children, adolescents, and young adults (24 and younger).

Stimulants

Amphetamine, d, (Dexedrine)

Starting Dose: 5 mg PO BID.

Titration: Increase by 5–10 mg PO BID each week.

Max Dose: 60 mg/day,

FDA Approval: ADHD ages 6 and up.

Common Side Effects: Insomnia, headache, exacerbation of tics, nervousness, irritability, overstimulation, tremor, dizziness, anorexia, dry mouth, nausea, diarrhea, constipation, sexual dysfunction long term.

Uncommon: *Psychotic episodes, seizures, palpitations, cardiovascular adverse effects.*

Monitoring: Assess for cardiac disease before initiation. Blood pressure and heart rate should be monitored regularly. Monitor height and weight in children.

Contraindications: Extreme anxiety, motor tics, taking an MAO-I, patient has history of arteriosclerosis, cardiovascular disease, severe hypertension, glaucoma, structural cardiac abnormalities, cardiomyopathy, serious heart arrhythmias, or CAD.

Black Box Warning: High abuse potential.

Amphetamine, d, l (Adderall, Adderall XR)

Starting Dose: 5 mg PO BID. Extended Release: 12.5 mg PO upon waking.

Titration: Increase by 5–10 mg PO BID each week. Extended Release: Increase by 12.5 mg PO daily every week.

Max Dose: 40 mg/day. Extended Release: 50 mg/day.

FDA Approval: ADHD ages 6 and up. Narcolepsy in patients ages 6 and up. Exogenous obesity in ages 12 and up.

Common Side Effects: Insomnia, headache, exacerbation of tics, nervousness, irritability, overstimulation, tremor, dizziness, anorexia, dry mouth, nausea, diarrhea, constipation, sexual dysfunction long term.

Uncommon: *Psychotic episodes, seizures, palpitations, cardiovascular adverse effects.*

Monitoring: Assess for cardiac disease before initiation. Blood pressure and heart rate should be monitored regularly. Monitor height and weight in children.

Contraindications: Extreme anxiety, motor tics, taking an MAO-I, patient has history of arteriosclerosis, cardiovascular disease, severe hypertension, glaucoma, structural cardiac abnormalities, cardiomyopathy, serious heart arrhythmias, or CAD.

Black Box Warning: High abuse potential.

Lisdexamfetamine (Vyvanse)

Starting Dose: 30 mg PO daily.

Titration: Increase 10–20 mg PO daily every week.

Max Dose: 70 mg/day.

FDA Approval: ADHD ages 6 and up. Binge eating disorder.

Common Side Effects: Fatigue, sleepiness, insomnia, irritability, headache, decreased appetite, nausea, vomiting, dry mouth, constipation, increased heart rate and blood pressure,

Uncommon: *Psychotic episodes, seizures, palpitations, tachycardia, hypertension, cardiovascular adverse effects.*

Rare: *Activation of hypomania.*

Monitoring: Blood pressure at initiation, after dose increase, and periodically throughout treatment.

Contraindications: Taking MAO-I inhibitor, history of pheochromocytoma, angle-closure glaucoma, hyperthyroidism, and severe cardiovascular disorder.

Pearl: Taper to avoid withdrawal effects.

Black Box Warning: High abuse potential.

Methylphenidate d (Focalin)

Starting Dose: 2.5 mg PO BID,

Titration: Increase by 2.5–5 mg/day every week.

Max Dose: 10 mg BID.

FDA Approval: ADHD ages 6–17.

Common Side Effects: Insomnia, headache, exacerbation of tics, nervousness, irritability, overstimulation, tremor, dizziness, anorexia, dry mouth, nausea.

Uncommon: *Psychotic episodes*, *seizures*, *palpitations*, *priapism*, and *cardiovascular adverse effects.*

Monitoring: Assess for cardiac disease before initiation. Blood pressure and heart rate should be monitored regularly. Monitor height and weight in children.

Contraindications: Extreme anxiety, motor tics, taking an MAO-I, cardiovascular disease, glaucoma, structural cardiac abnormalities, cardiomyopathy, serious heart arrhythmias, or CAD.

Black Box Warning: High abuse potential.

Methylphenidate d Extended Release Capsules (Focalin XR)

Starting Dose: 10 mg PO daily,

Titration: Increase by 10 mg/day, after 1 week.

Max Dose: 40 mg daily.

FDA Approval: ADHD ages 6–17. ADHD in adults.

Common Side Effects: Insomnia, headache, exacerbation of tics, nervousness, irritability, overstimulation, tremor, dizziness, anorexia, dry mouth, nausea.

Uncommon: *Psychotic episodes, seizures, palpitations, priapism, and cardiovascular adverse effects.*

Monitoring: Assess for cardiac disease before initiation. Blood pressure and heart rate should be monitored regularly. Monitor height and weight in children.

Contraindications: Extreme anxiety, motor tics, taking an MAO-I, cardiovascular disease, glaucoma, structural cardiac abnormalities, cardiomyopathy, serious heart arrhythmias, or CAD.

Black Box Warning: High abuse potential.

Methylphenidate d, l (Ritalin)

Starting Dose: 5 mg PO in the am and at lunch,

Titration: Increase by 5–10 mg every week.

Max Dose: 60 mg BID.

FDA Approval: ADHD. Narcolepsy.

Common Side Effects: Insomnia, headache, exacerbation of tics, nervousness, irritability, overstimulation, tremor, dizziness, anorexia, dry mouth, nausea.

Uncommon: *Psychotic episodes, seizures, palpitations, priapism,* and *cardiovascular adverse effects*.

Monitoring: Assess for cardiac disease before initiation. Blood pressure and heart rate should be monitored regularly. Monitor height and weight in children.

Contraindications: Extreme anxiety, motor tics, taking an MAO-I, cardiovascular disease, glaucoma, structural cardiac abnormalities, cardiomyopathy, serious heart arrhythmias, or CAD.

Black Box Warning: High abuse potential.

Methylphenidate d, l (Concerta)

Starting Dose: 18 mg PO daily.

Titration: Increase by 18 mg every week.

Max Dose: 72 mg BID.

FDA Approval: ADHD. Narcolepsy.

Common Side Effects: Insomnia, headache, exacerbation of tics, nervousness, irritability, overstimulation, tremor, dizziness, anorexia, dry mouth, nausea.

Uncommon: *Psychotic episodes, seizures, palpitations, priapism*, and *cardiovascular adverse effects.*

Monitoring: Assess for cardiac disease before initiation. Blood pressure and heart rate should be monitored regularly. Monitor height and weight in children.

Contraindications: Extreme anxiety, motor tics, taking an MAO-I, cardiovascular disease, glaucoma, structural cardiac abnormalities, cardiomyopathy, serious heart arrhythmias, or CAD.

Black Box Warning: High abuse potential.

Methylphenidate HCL (Jornay PM)

Starting Dose: 20 mg PO nightly.

Titration: Increase by 20 mg every week.

Max Dose: 100 mg daily.

FDA Approval: ADHD in 6 years and older.

Common Side Effects: Insomnia, headache, exacerbation of tics, nervousness, irritability, overstimulation, tremor, dizziness, anorexia, dry mouth, nausea.

Uncommon: *Psychotic episodes, seizures, palpitations, priapism*, and *cardiovascular adverse effects*.

Monitoring: Assess for cardiac disease before initiation. Blood pressure and heart rate should be monitored regularly. Monitor height and weight in children.

Contraindications: Extreme anxiety, motor tics, taking an MAO-I, cardiovascular disease, glaucoma, structural cardiac abnormalities, cardiomyopathy, serious heart arrhythmias, or CAD.

Black Box Warning: High abuse potential.

Serdexmethylphenidate (Azstarys)

Starting Dose: 39.5 mg/7.8 mg daily.

Titration: Increase to 52.3 mg/10.4 mg daily after 7 days.

Max Dose: 52.3 mg/10.4 mg.

FDA Approval: ADHD for over 6 years of age.

Common Side Effects: Insomnia, headache, exacerbation of tics, nervousness, irritability, overstimulation, tremor, dizziness, anorexia, dry mouth, nausea.

Uncommon: *Psychotic episodes, seizures, palpitations, priapism,* and *cardiovascular adverse effects.*

Monitoring: Assess for cardiac disease before initiation. Blood pressure and heart rate should be monitored regularly. Monitor height and weight in children.

Contraindications: Extreme anxiety, motor tics, taking an MAO-I, cardiovascular disease, glaucoma, structural cardiac abnormalities, cardiomyopathy, serious heart arrhythmias, or CAD.

Black Box Warning: High abuse potential.

Substance Abuse Medications

Acamprosate (Campral)

Starting Dose: 666 mg PO three times a day.

Titration: Not required.

Max Dose: 666 mg PO three times a day.

FDA Approval: Maintenance of alcohol abstinence.

Common Side Effects: Diarrhea, nausea, anxiety, depression, *suicidality.*

Monitoring: None.

Contraindication: Renal impairment.

Pearl: Best used for alcohol abstinence not goal of reduced drinking.

Black Box Warning: Liver damage or hepatitis (hepatotoxicity)

Bupropion SR (Wellbutrin SR)

Starting Dose: 150 mg PO daily.

Titration: Increase by 150 mg PO daily after 3 days.

Max Dose: 300 mg PO daily.

FDA Approval: MDD, seasonal affective disorder, nicotine addiction (standard release).

Common Side Effects: Dry mouth, GI upset, insomnia, dizziness, headache, agitation, anxiety, tremor, sweating, weight loss, anorexia, myalgia, tinnitus, rash, hypertension.

Rare: *Seizures, Stevens-Johnson syndrome has been reported, induction of mania, and activation of suicidal ideation in those under 24.*

Monitoring: PHQ-9.

PEARL: XL only requires once a day dosing, making it the preferred preparation. Can be given with other antidepressants to help with sexual side effects.

Contraindicated: Patients with current or prior diagnosis of bulimia or anorexia nervosa. Patients with a history of seizures. If patient is abruptly quitting alcohol, sedative use, or anticonvulsant medication. If patient has had a recent head injury or has a nervous system tumor.

Disulfiram (Antabuse)

Starting Dose: 250 mg PO daily.

Titration: 125–250 mg PO daily.

Max Dose: 500 mg PO daily.

FDA Approval: Maintenance of alcohol abstinence.

Common Side Effects: Flushing, headache, tachycardia, nausea, vomiting if consuming alcohol, metallic taste dermatitis, sedation,

Uncommon: *Myocardial infarction, congestive heart failure, respiratory depression, hepatotoxicity* if alcohol is consumed.

Monitoring: Baseline liver function test and then periodic testing afterwards.

Contraindications: If patient is intoxicated, drank within last 12 h, psychosis, cardiovascular disease, on certain medications: metronidazole, amprenavir, ritonavir, or sertraline.

Pearl: Do not take disulfiram until at least 12 h after drinking.

Black Box Warning: Never administer if alcohol intoxication or without patient's full consent.

Naltrexone (Revia/Vivitrol)

Starting Dose: 50 mg PO daily. 380 mg every 4 weeks for injection (Vivitrol).

Titration: None.

Max Dose: 50 mg PO daily. 380 mg every 4 weeks for injection.

FDA Approval: Alcohol dependence, blockade effects of exogenously administered opioids, Relapse prevention of opioid dependence.

Common Side Effects: Nausea, vomiting, decreased appetite, dizziness, injection site reactions, dysphoria, and anxiety.

Uncommon: *Eosinophilic pneumonia, hepatocellular injury at high doses, severe injection site reactions requiring surgery.*

Monitoring: Liver function prior to initiating treatment. Urine drug screen in certain cases to make sure no opioids in system.

Contraindication: Patients receiving opioid analgesics, current physiologic opioid dependence. In acute opioid withdrawal, patients who have failed the naloxone challenge test or have a positive urine screen for opioids, hypersensitivity to naltrexone, polylactide-co-glycolide (PLG), carboxymethylcellulose, or any other components of the diluent.

Pearl: Patients should have medical alert bracelet for naltrexone use.

Black box warning: Liver damage or hepatitis (hepatotoxicity).

Nicotine Transmucosal (Nicorette Gum)

First cigarette more than 30 min after awakening: 2 mg by mouth every 1–2 h × 6 weeks, then every 2–4 h × 3 weeks, then every 4–8 h × 3 weeks.

First cigarette less than 30 min after awakening: 4 mg by mouth every 1–2 h × 6 weeks, then every 2–4 h × 3 weeks, then every 4–8 h × 3 weeks.

Max Dose: 24 mg.

FDA Approval: Nicotine dependence.

Common Side Effects: Withdrawal symptoms, palpitations, hypertension, nausea, hiccups, flatulence, cough, sore throat, paresthesia, arthralgia, URI symptoms.

Uncommon: *Nicotine dependence transference.*

Contraindications: Severe arrhythmia, acute MI within last 2 weeks, worsening/severe angina.

PEARL: Avoid food or drink within 15 min before or after use.

Nicotine Transdermal (Nicoderm CQ)

Greater than 10 cigarettes per day: 21 mg transdermal daily × 6 weeks, then 14 mg/day × 2 weeks, then apply 7 mg patch daily × 2 weeks. Start on day 1 of quitting.

Less than 10 cigarettes per day: Apply 14 mg patch daily × 6 weeks, then apply 7 mg patch daily × 2 weeks. Start on day 1 of quitting.

FDA Approval: Nicotine addiction and dependence.

Common Side Effects: Local skin reaction and edema, rash, withdrawal symptoms, headache, palpitations, tachycardia, hypertension, nausea, hiccups, constipation, flatulence, diarrhea, paresthesia, arthralgia, chest discomfort, insomnia, and abnormal dreams.

Uncommon: *Nicotine dependence transference, hypersensitivity reaction.*

Contraindications: Severe arrhythmia, acute MI within last 2 weeks, worsening/severe angina.

Topiramate (Topamax)

Starting Dose: 25 mg PO nightly.

Titration: Increase by 25 mg PO nightly every 7 days.

Max Dose: 400 mg

FDA Approval: Seizures, migraine prophylaxis, chronic weight management.

Common Side Effects: Sedation, asthenia, dizziness, ataxia, paresthesia, nystagmus, nervousness, tremor, nausea, appetite loss, weight loss, blurred/double vision, confusion, memory problems, mood problems, fatigue, and taste disturbances.

Uncommon: *Metabolic ketoacidosis*, kidney stones, *hyperammonemia*, *rare SJS or purpura*, *hyperthermia*, *rare activation of suicidality*.

Monitoring: Baseline serum bicarbonate and then periodically, checking for hyperchloremic, non-anion gap metabolic acidosis.

Contraindications: Within a 6 h window of alcohol use, patients with metabolic acidosis while on metformin.

Pearl: Has been shown to reduce number of episodes of binge-drinking.

Varenicline (Chantix)

Starting Dose: 0.5 mg PO daily.

Titration: After 3 days increase to 0.5 mg PO BID and after 4 days increase to 1 mg PO BID.

Max Dose: 1 mg PO BID.

FDA Approval: Nicotine addiction and dependence.

Common Side Effects: Nausea, vomiting, constipation, flatulence, insomnia, headache, abnormal dreams,

Rare: *Agitation, depressed mood, suicidal ideation and behavior, seizures.*

PEARL: Take with meal and full glass of water. Pt should start treatment 1 week prior to quit date or quit smoking between 8 and 35 days of starting Chantix. Depression should be well controlled before starting.

Index

B. Floyd, T. Kane, *The Clinician's Guide to Common Psychiatric Disorders*, https://doi.org/10.1007/978-3-031-67958-2

F

G

H

I

L

MIX
Papier aus verantwortungsvollen Quellen
Paper from responsible sources
FSC® C105338

If you have any concerns about our products,
you can contact us on
ProductSafety@springernature.com

In case Publisher is established outside the EU,
the EU authorized representative is:
Springer Nature Customer Service Center GmbH
Europaplatz 3, 69115 Heidelberg, Germany

Printed by Libri Plureos GmbH
in Hamburg, Germany